Blood a
Transp

MW00984857

Blood and Marrow Transplant Handbook

Comprehensive Guide for Patient Care

Richard T. Maziarz, MD
Portland, Oregon, USA

Susan Slater, MN, FNP-BC
Portland, Oregon, USA

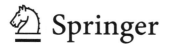

Editors
Richard T. Maziarz, MD
Center for Hematologic
  Malignancies
Adult Blood and Marrow Stem
  Cell Transplant Program
Knight Cancer Institute
Oregon Health & Science
  University
Portland, OR 97239, USA

Susan Slater, MN, FNP-BC
Center for Hematologic
  Malignancies
Adult Blood and Marrow Stem
  Cell Transplant Program
Knight Cancer Institute
Oregon Health & Science
  University
Portland, OR 97239, USA

ISBN 978-1-4419-7505-8   e-ISBN 978-1-4419-7506-5
DOI 10.1007/978-1-4419-7506-5
Springer New York Dordrecht Heidelberg London

Springer is part of Springer Science+Business Media (www.springer.com)

Preface and Acknowledgments

Hematopoietic stem cell transplantation has experienced a dramatic increase of activity over the past decade with a continued marked escalation of procedures projected over the next ten to fifteen years. This expansion is not only a reflection of an ever changing field with increasing demand but also the pursuit of innovation that contributes to continued improved outcomes with less risk of adverse events or deleterious long-term consequences for the transplant patient population. Cell therapy is a dynamic field. It requires multi-specialty input for the management of these complex patients. In the past, transplantation was the sole responsibility of a few academic centers, and information resided within the hands of a few individuals. However, with the dissemination of technology and the ongoing proliferation of these procedures, there has been an obligatory need for the development of tools to provide standard guidelines and algorithms for the management of patients.

Most institutions have established their own set of guidelines and recommendations designed for consensus management as patients are in constant need of shared care. As new workforce demands have emerged, there have been changes in the workplace with recent predictions of a marked shortage of transplant physicians. As an alternative, more non-physician providers are being recruited to this field to provide day-to-day care of the transplant patient. In light of these changes, it becomes imperative to provide detailed and shared consensus guidelines to ensure the best and most predictable outcomes of our patients can be achieved.

This guide to patient management is the product of fifteen years of evolution of patient care at our institution. Wherever possible, the information herein has been altered to reflect the multiple options that exist for treatment of various conditions. However, *it is not meant to define the exact care pathway for all patients*. Rather, we have provided a practical set of guidelines that can be shared across institutions. This effort is our contribution to the workforce shortage for transplant physicians. By providing an easy-to-use manual that covers the basics of care of the stem cell transplant patient which can be utilized to educate physician assistants, nurse practitioners, residents, post-doctoral fellows, and other hospitalists that may be recruited to the day-to-day care of the patient, we have achieved our goal. We recognize that this pocket guide is a work in progress, and we anticipate that as time passes, even potentially quite quickly, a new set of guidelines will need to be generated.

We recognize that this manual is incomplete. We do not discuss graft engineering to any great degree. We are not addressing the nuances of cord blood transplantation. We are not considering haplo-identical transplantation or other therapies that remain in clinical trial development and may emerge soon into the clinical arena. Nor are we talking about regeneration medicine, its futures, and its overlap with hematopoietic stem cell transplantation. Rather, we provide information about standards of care and assimilate knowledge gained from others.

The work presented within this volume represents not the work of a few, but the work of many. A number of our authors were members of the team that helped create our institution-specific consensus guidelines. We have also recruited new members to assist in generating these ever changing set of standards. We wish to thank the many contributors, as well as our mentors and colleagues who have inspired us to pursue this field and who have provided us with the energy to make this contribution. We would like to thank Thomas Thomas for his assistance in the preparation of this manual. We specifically acknowledge the work of Florence Seelig, Peter Curtin, Mark Brunvand, Kamar Godder, Gerald Segal, and the late Keith Hansen among many of our former team members. Their contributions to our program cannot be underestimated. In addition, we thank our team of dedicated nurses, social workers, CMAs, CNAs, physical therapists, nutrition specialists, and all providers that are present at the patients' bedside. We also thank our collaborating community partners: referring physicians, mid-level providers, and nurse coordinators. Through collaboration and shared information, we hope to assure the best outcome of our patients as they return to their communities across the country.

Editors, 2011   Richard T. Maziarz, MD
                                                 Susan Slater, MN, FNP-BC

Contents

Part I   The Nuts and Bolts of Stem Cell Transplant

1   **Overview of Hematopoietic Stem Cell Transplantation** 3
    Richard T. Maziarz

2   **The Business of Cellular Therapy and Hematopoietic Stem Cell Transplantation** . . . 9
    Peggy Appel and Richard T. Maziarz

3   **Stem Cell Sources** 21
    Jose Leis

4   **Pre-transplant Evaluation** 27
    Andy Chen

5   **Conditioning Regimens** 39
    Joseph Bubalo

6   **Supportive Care** 51
    Bryon Allen

7   **Nutrition** 63
    Stacey Evert

8   **Infection Prophylaxis** 71
    Lynne Strasfeld

9   **Graft-Versus-Host Disease Prophylaxis** 83
    Erin Corella

10 **Transfusion Medicine** 101
    James Gajewski and Susan Slater

11 **Antithrombotic Guidelines** 111
    Thomas DeLoughery

12 **Engraftment** 119
    Sara Murray

13 **Follow-Up Care** 125
    Carol Jacoby

Part II   Transplant Complications

14   **Infectious Complications**   143
     Lynne Strasfeld

15   **Acute Graft-Versus-Host Disease**   167
     Susan Slater

16   **Chronic Graft-Versus-Host Disease**   189
     Richard T. Maziarz and Farnoush Abar

17   **Oral Complications**   213
     Kimberly Brennan Tyler

18   **Gastrointestinal Complications**   223
     Eneida Nemecek

19   **Pulmonary Complications**   233
     Tarek Eid and Alan F. Barker

20   **Cardiovascular Complications**   245
     Christopher Greenman

21   **Acute Kidney Injury**   253
     Anuja Mittalhenkle

22   **Thrombotic Microangiopathies**   261
     Thomas DeLoughery

23   **Graft Failure**   265
     Gabrielle Meyers

24   **Post-transplant Relapse**   271
     Richard T. Maziarz and Susan Slater

25   **Palliative Care**   277
     Mary Denise Smith and Amy Guthrie

26   **Survivorship**   281
     Lisa Hansen and Brandon Hayes-Lattin

Appendices   297
Index   309

Contributors

Farnoush Abar, MD
Center for Hematologic Malignancies, Adult Blood and Marrow Stem Cell Transplant Program, Oregon Health and Science University, Portland, OR, USA

Bryon Allen, MSN, FNP-BC
Center for Hematologic Malignancies, Adult Blood and Marrow Stem Cell Transplant Program, Oregon Health and Science University, Portland, OR, USA

Peggy Appel, MHA
Northwest Marrow Transplant Program, Oregon Health and Science University, Portland, OR, USA

Alan F. Barker, MD
Pulmonary and Critical Care Medicine, Oregon Health and Science University, Portland, OR, USA

Joseph Bubalo, Pharm D, BCPS, BCOP
Clinical Operations Manager and Oncology Clinical Pharmacist, Pharmacy Services, Oregon Health and Science University, Portland, OR, USA

Andy Chen, MD, PhD
Center for Hematologic Malignancies, Adult Blood and Marrow Stem Cell Transplant Program, Oregon Health and Science University, Portland, OR, USA

Erin Corella, Pharm D, BCPS, BCOP
Pharmacy Services, Oregon Health and Science University, Portland, OR, USA

Thomas DeLoughery, MD
Divisions of Hematology/Oncology and Laboratory Medicine, Oregon Health and Science University, Portland, OR, USA

Tarek Eid, MD
Pulmonary and Critical Care Medicine, Oregon Health and Science University, Portland, OR, USA

Stacey Evert, RD, CSO, LD
Bone Marrow Transplant/Oncology Dietitian, Food and
Nutrition Services, Oregon Health and Science University,
Portland, OR, USA

James Gajewski, MD
Center for Hematologic Malignancies, Adult Blood and
Marrow Stem Cell Transplant Program, Oregon Health and
Science University, Portland, OR, USA

Christopher Greenman, MD
Department of Medicine, Oregon Health and Science
University, Portland, OR, USA

Amy Guthrie, MSN, CNS, ACHPN
Palliative Medicine/Comfort Care Team, Oregon Health and
Science University, Portland, OR, USA

Lisa Hansen, RN, MS, CNS, AOCN
Autologous Stem Cell Transplantation, Legacy Good
Samaritan Hospital, Portland, OR, USA

Brandon Hayes-Lattin, MD
Center for Hematologic Malignancies, Adult Blood and
Marrow Stem Cell Transplant Program, Oregon Health and
Science University, Portland, OR, USA

Carol Jacoby, MSN, ACNP-BC
Center for Hematologic Malignancies, Adult Blood and
Marrow Stem Cell Transplant Program, Oregon Health and
Science University, Portland, OR, USA

Jose Leis, MD, PhD
Adult Blood and Marrow Transplant Program, Mayo Clinic,
Phoenix, AZ, USA

Richard T. Maziarz, MD
Center for Hematologic Malignancies, Adult Blood and
Marrow Stem Cell Transplant Program, Oregon Health and
Science University, Portland, OR, USA

Gabrielle Meyers, MD
Center for Hematologic Malignancies, Adult Blood and
Marrow Stem Cell Transplant Program, Oregon Health and
Science University, Portland, OR, USA

Anuja Mittalhenkle, MD
Division of Nephrology and Hypertension, Oregon Health and
Science University, Portland, OR, USA

Sara Murray, BS, DAS
Center for Hematologic Malignancies, Adult Blood and
Marrow Stem Cell Transplant Program, Oregon Health and
Science University, Portland, OR, USA

Eneida Nemecek, MD
Pediatric Blood and Marrow Transplantation, Doernbecher
Children's Hospital, Portland, OR, USA

Susan Slater, MN, FNP-BC
Center for Hematologic Malignancies, Adult Blood and
Marrow Stem Cell Transplant Program, Oregon Health and
Science University, Portland, OR, USA

Mary Denise Smith, MSN, CNS, ACHPN
Palliative Medicine/Comfort Care Team, Oregon Health and
Science University, Portland, OR, USA

Lynne Strasfeld, MD
Department of Infectious Disease, Oregon Health and Science
University, Portland, OR, USA

Kimberly Brennan Tyler, MSN, ANP-BC
Center for Hematologic Malignancies, Adult Blood and
Marrow Stem Cell Transplant Program, Oregon Health and
Science University, Portland, OR, USA

PART I

The Nuts and Bolts of Stem Cell Transplant

CHAPTER I
Overview of Hematopoietic Stem Cell Transplantation

Richard T. Maziarz

Hematopoietic stem cell transplantation (HSCT) has evolved over the past 50–60 years to become the standard of care procedure for many disorders. Advances in immunogenetics and immunobiology, conditioning regimens, disease characterization and risk stratification, immune suppression, antimicrobials, and other types of supportive care have made this expansion possible. Some of the earliest work contributed to the first successful bone marrow transplant, performed in a young child with immune deficiency syndrome in 1968. Approximately 15 years later, the graft-versus-leukemia response was recognized as overlapping with the development of graft-versus-host disease (GvHD). In the early 1980s, bone marrow transplantation was no longer considered experimental, but as the standard of care for a variety of disorders including acute leukemia and aplastic anemia. With this recognition, the incidence of this procedure rapidly increased to the current state where over 50,000 procedures are performed worldwide each year as estimated by the Center for International Blood and Marrow Transplant Research (CIBMTR).

I.I THE LANGUAGE OF TRANSPLANTATION

HSCT can often appear daunting to newcomers to the field as a consequence of the intensity of treatments administered to patients, the breadth of medical knowledge required by the clinical transplantation specialist, and the specialized language used by the HSCT expert. A partial list of definitions is provided to assist the newcomer.

R.T. Maziarz, S. Slater (eds.), *Blood and Marrow Transplant Handbook*, DOI 10.1007/978-1-4419-7506-5_1, © Springer Science+Business Media, LLC 2011

1. *Hematopoietic stem cell*: A bone marrow-derived stem cell with the capacity for self-renewal and the ability to generate downstream mature products of red cells, white blood cells, and platelets. By definition, a transplantable product
2. *Autologous*: Cells derived or obtained from the afflicted individual
3. *Allogeneic*: Cells derived or obtained from another individual
4. *Syngeneic*: Cells derived or obtained from an identical twin
5. *HLA*: Histocompatibility locus antigen
   a. HLA Class I: Gene products of HLA A, B, C, universally expressed on the surface of all cells of an individual (with some specific exceptions, e.g., trophoblast tissue); the class of histocompatibility molecules that present cellular peptides to CD8 T-cell effectors
   b. HLA Class II: Gene products of HLA DR, DP, DQ, cell surface expression normally limited to lymphohematopoietic tissues but can be induced on many tissues after inflammatory cytokine exposure; the class of histocompatibility molecules that present cellular peptides to CD4 T-cell effectors
   c. Antigen: Any molecule that is recognized and bound by immunoglobulin or T-cell receptors; in immunogenetics, this term is often interchangeably used to describe a particular HLA molecule
   d. Allele: Molecular variants of a single gene
   e. Antigenic determinant/epitope: The specific part of an antigen bound by immunoglobulin or T-cell receptor
6. *MHC*: Major histocompatibility complex. The collection of genes located on human chromosome 6 that encode the polymorphic proteins involved in antigen presentation to T cells; the regulators of the cellular immune response
7. *Haplotype*: The location of a linked set of polymorphic HLA genes on a single chromosome; all cells, other than the germ cells of an individual, express two haplotypes, each inherited from a single parent
8. *Haploidentical*: The circumstance in transplantation in which there is a partial or complete mismatch at a single HLA locus between two individuals
9. *CD34*: A surface marker of the earliest progenitors and stem cell pools. Clinical exploitation has been achieved using this molecule in determining if adequate numbers of transplantable stem cells are obtained prior to a procedure

10. *Bone marrow harvest*: The procedure through which donor stem cells are collected directly from the bone marrow cavity

11. *Peripheral blood stem cell collection (apheresis)*: The procedure by which stem cells are mobilized directly into the blood of the donor for harvesting by leukapheresis
    a. Mobilization: The act of enhancing the movement of stem cells from their microenvironment niche into circulation; usually performed with growth factor or growth factor plus chemotherapy exposure

12. *Conditioning*: The euphemistic term for the chemotherapy- or radiation-based preparation of the host prior to the transplant, the goals of which include immune suppression and myelosuppression

13. *Myeloablative*: Conditioning regimens designed to eliminate all host stem cells

14. *Non-myeloablative*: Conditioning focused on immune suppression and establishment of donor chimerism without dose intensity enough to destroy all residual host stem cells
    a. Chimerism: the establishment of donor cells within another recipient; can be partial or complete

15. *Reduced intensity transplantation*: A blanket term for any degree of conditioning that is less intense than traditionally defined maximal myeloablative conditioning

16. *CIBMTR*: Center for International Blood and Marrow Transplant Registry, the registry of >400 transplant centers worldwide that contribute outcomes data to a central data repository for analysis

17. *NMDP*: National Marrow Donor Program. An American organization focused on facilitating unrelated donor and cord blood transplant procedures

18. *ASBMT*: American Society for Blood and Marrow Transplantation. An international professional association that promotes the blood and marrow transplantation field

19. *BMT CTN*: Blood and Marrow Transplant Clinical Trials Network. National Heart, Lung, and Blood Institute (NHLBI) and National Cancer Institute (NCI)-sponsored intergroup focused on the development of clinical trials in the hematopoietic stem cell transplantation arena

20. *NCI CTC*: National Cancer Institute Common Toxicity Criteria. A widely accepted criteria for assessing severity of adverse events. Its utilization allows for overcoming institutional variation in reporting and for comparative outcomes research to be performed

21. *EBMT*: The European Group for Blood and Marrow Transplantation. An organization based in Europe that promotes cooperative studies and collects transplant outcome data from multiple European and Eurasian countries
22. *WMDA*: The World Marrow Donor Foundation. An international organization focused on donor safety, stem cell accessibility, and generation of standard practices for the exchange of hematopoietic stem cells for clinical transplantation worldwide

1.2 RESEARCH EFFORTS IN HSCT

The success of HSCT has had its origins in the research laboratories and clinical research units at many institutions. However, it is also recognized that there is a continued need for ongoing research. Much of the material within this guidebook reflects established standards of care of management in the HSCT patient. However, the field demands constant efforts for improvement. There are many areas of active research including new conditioning regimens, new immune-suppressive approaches, vaccines (both prior to and after transplantation) focused at infectious pathogens as well as the primary malignancy, T regulatory cells, new indications such as autoimmune disease or sickle cell disease, applications of natural killer cells, novel stem cell mobilization ages, and continued improvement in supportive care. Recently, the ASBMT published a set of research priorities to assist in the focus of attention to those fields that are most likely to lead to continued development of hematopoietic cellular therapy. These include

1. Stem cell biology
   a. Cell manipulation
   b. Stem cell sources
   c. Inducible pluripotent stem cells
   d. Cancer stem cells
2. Tumor relapse
   a. Prevention of and therapy for post-transplant relapse
   b. Immunotherapy with T-cell and dendritic cells
3. Graft-versus-host disease
   a. Separation of GvHD and graft-versus-tumor effects
   b. Immune reconstitution in GvHD
   c. Markers predicting GvHD
   d. Role of regulatory T cells
4. Applying new technology to HSCT

   a. Genomics
   b. Proteomics
   c. Imaging
   d. Markers of immunologic recovery
   e. Pharmacogenomics
5. Expanded indications for HSCT
   a. Solid tumors
   b. Regenerative medicine
   c. Autoimmune disease
   d. Response to bioterrorism in radiation accidents
6. Survivorship
   a. Long-term complications
   b. Longevity
   c. Quality of life
7. Transplants in older patients
   a. Biology of aging
   b. Indications for transplant
   c. Outcomes and quality of life
8. Improving current use of HSCT
   a. Graft sources
   b. Conditioning intensity
   c. Cost-effectiveness

1.3 HORIZONS/CHALLENGES

HSCT remains an expanding field. As described briefly above, these technologies have been applied to thousands of people within dozens of countries. The success of the varied research initiatives will extend these applications to a greater degree. Currently, the NMDP projects facilitation of double the number of unrelated transplant procedures over the next 5 years, from current levels of nearly 5,000 annually to over 10,000 by 2015. This growth has been multifactorial and is impacted by broader indications, improved supportive care, changing age demographics with increased incidence of cancers reported, and improved survivorship of patients with cardiovascular disease.

With these predictions, one must also be aware that the development of molecular therapeutics may lead to an alternate future. Much of cancer therapy research today is focused on the "personalized" medicine approach in which small molecules that target the multiple signaling pathways might convert life-threatening malignancies to truly chronic diseases. The impact of imatinib mesylate (Gleevec®) on transplantation for chronic myeloid leukemia is a prime example.

However, we must be aware that the increased numbers of patients undergoing transplantation, as well as the observed improvement in survival, will lead to a greater demand for specialists in the field of HSCT. Not only are the patients who undergo transplantation in need of specialized providers but also the rapidly expanding population of survivors, particularly those with chronic graft-versus-host disease, has difficulty finding a medical home with their primary care providers or referring medical oncologists.

A recent analysis suggests that within the very near future there will be a significant shortfall in physicians trained and focused on the care of HSCT patients. Thus, new paradigms must be developed for the delivery of care to the HSCT survivor, including expansion of the non-physician provider workforce of physician assistants and nurse practitioners, as well as active recruitment of new trainees in the field of hematology and medical oncology. Most importantly, training programs and generation of tools must be established for a new specialty of primary care providers focused on delivery of chronic care to the cancer survivor.

References

Deeg, H., DiPersio, J., Young, J., Maziarz, R., Perreault, C., Margolis, D., et al. (2009). ASBMT policy statement 2009 research priorities. *Biol Blood Marrow Transplant*, 15:1489–1491.

Gajewski, J., LeMaistre, F., Silver, S., Lill, M., Selby, G., Horowitz, M., et al. (2009). Impending challenges in the hematopoietic stem cell transplantation physician workforce. *Biol Blood Marrow Transplant*, 15:1493–1501.

Giralt, S., Arora, M., Goldman, J., Lee, S., Maziarz, R., McCarthy, P., et al. (2007). Impact of imatinib therapy on the use of allogeneic haematopoietic progenitor cell transplantation for the treatment of chronic myeloid leukaemia. *Br J Haematol*, 137:461–467.

CHAPTER 2

The Business of Cellular Therapy and Hematopoietic Stem Cell Transplantation

Peggy Appel and Richard T. Maziarz

Hematopoietic stem cell transplant (HSCT) is a complex process that is associated with a heavy demand for resources and need for multispecialty teams. The first transplant procedures were performed over 40 years ago. There has been a dramatic increase in the number of procedures performed over the past 10 years (Fig. 2.1).

National Marrow Donor Program (NMDP) projections for growth in unrelated donor transplants are significant with an expected doubling of facilitated transplants projected at 10,000 by the year 2015. These projections can be frightening, but recent analysis of US hospitalization utilization indicates that in the past 5 years, there has already been a doubling of activity. Bone marrow transplant ranked highest among the commonly performed procedures with the most rapidly increasing hospital inpatient costs from 2004 to 2007, with a percentage change in total costs of 84.9% and a percentage change in total hospital stays of 51.3%. In the breakdown, it was observed that specifically inpatient costs for Medicare covered stays increased 90.4% and costs for private payer insured stays increased 100.6% during this period (Table 2.1).

In the settings of increasing demand and increasing cost of technologies, it is critical for providers and hospital systems to assure that contractual arrangements with payers have sufficient complexity to support the provision of the best care while protecting from excessive financial risk, resulting in financial stability of the transplant program.

R.T. Maziarz, S. Slater (eds.), *Blood and Marrow Transplant Handbook*, DOI 10.1007/978-1-4419-7506-5_2, © Springer Science+Business Media, LLC 2011

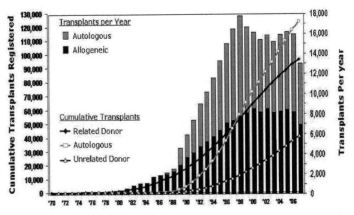

FIG. 2.1. Annual and cumulative transplant procedures reported to the CIBMTR

2.1 COMPLEXITY OF CARE

Hospitals and payers alike typically wish to "carve out" HSCT services from general medical services contracts. Due to the complexity of care delivered, variability in patient care requirements, and potential risk of need for catastrophic care, HSCT services are often divided into phases for the purposes of authorization and reimbursement methodologies. These phases may encompass consultation, evaluation, transplant, and post-transplant.

2.2 PHASES

1. Transplant evaluation
    a. Begins when a new patient is referred for transplant evaluation
    b. Ends when patient is approved as a transplant candidate
    c. Inclusions
        i. Physician and clinic charges for consultation and physical exam
        ii. Lab tests
        iii. Radiology studies
        iv. Psychiatric evaluation
        v. Dental evaluation
        vi. Patient and donor HLA typing
        vii. Donor infectious disease testing

TABLE 2.1. Commonly performed procedures with the most rapidly increasing hospital inpatient costs, 2004–2007

Principal procedure category	Total costs (2007)	Total hospital stays (2007)	Percentage change	
			Total costs (2004–2007) (%)	Total hospital stays (2004–2007) (%)
Bone marrow transplant	$1,282,645,000	15,100	84.9	51.3
Open prostatectomy	$1,032,016,000	88,500	68.6	40.8
Aortic resection; replacement or anastomosis	$1,872,908,000	61,600	38.5	31.9
Cancer chemotherapy	$2,616,504,000	187,400	33.2	14.2
Spinal fusion	$8,863,922,000	350,700	29.5	15.6
Lobectomy or pneumonectomy	$1,757,748,000	81,400	29.2	24.9
Incision and drainage, skin and subcutaneous tissue	$1,108,187,000	158,600	28.6	31.5
Arthroplasty knee	$9,217,740,000	605,200	27.5	25.7
Nephrotomy and nephrostomy	$682,609,000	38,600	25.3	11.7
Mastectomy	$660,173,000	70,100	23.8	3.6
Total for top 10 procedures[a]	$29,094,452,000	1,657,100	32.3	22.2

Source: AHRQ, Center for Delivery, Organization, and Markets, Healthcare Cost and Utilization Project, Nationwide Inpatient Sample, 2004 and 2007

[a] 2004 costs were adjusted to 2007 dollars using the overall Consumer Price Index

    d. Exclusions
      i. Non-transplant-related services
2. Pre-transplant
    a. Begins when a patient is identified as a transplant candidate
    b. Ends the day prior to the transplant admission
    c. Inclusions
      i. All inpatient and outpatient facility, professional, ancillary, and laboratory services related to routine surveillance of patient to assure maintenance of transplant-ready status
    d. Exclusions
      i. Disease-related services
3. Harvest/acquisition (typically included in pre-transplant phase or transplant phase)
    a. Inclusions
      i. Mobilization
      ii. Bone marrow or peripheral blood stem cell harvest
      iii. Acquisition charges for unrelated donor product procurement
      iv. Cell processing
4. Transplant stay
    a. Begins on the day of admission; or for outpatient transplants, with the initiation of preparative regimen
    b. Ends on the day of discharge; or for outpatient transplants, x number of days following stem cell infusion
    c. Inclusions
      i. All facility, professional, and ancillary charges
5. Post-transplant
    a. Begins on the day of discharge; or for outpatient transplants, x number of days following stem cell infusion
    b. Ends x number of days post-infusion or post-discharge
    c. Inclusions
      i. All transplant-related outpatient and inpatient facility and professional charges
      ii. Inpatient readmissions
    d. Exclusions
      i. Non-transplant-related services
6. Special circumstances
There are some HSCT-associated activities that require special arrangements or should be addressed separately from case rate provisions in contracts due to their unpredictability and/or variation in occurrence.
    a. Sequential transplants (pre-planned)

    b. Donor leukocyte infusions
    c. Re-transplants
    d. Reduced intensity transplants
    e. High-cost pharmacy items (e.g., plerixafor)

2.3 CONTRACTS AND REIMBURSEMENT STRATEGIES

If structured appropriately, contracts should reflect mutual exposure to financial risk.

    Reimbursement methodologies vary in the degree to which financial risk is shared.

1. Reimbursement methodologies
   a. Discount off charges – a flat percent discounting of billed charges
   b. Case rate – fixed fee that covers all transplant-related services for a specified period of time
   c. Global case rate – fixed fee that includes hospital and physician charges for a specified period of time; typically includes post-transplant care
2. Case rate and global case rate methodologies typically include provisions that protect the transplant center from financial risk. These provisions vary in the amount of financial protection they provide.
   a. Outlier days – per diem for each inpatient day in a defined post-infusion time period
   b. Outlier threshold – percentage of billed charges once a specified threshold beyond the case rate is reached
   c. Floor provision – at no time shall hospital be reimbursed less than $x\%$ of billed charges. This provision is usually used in tandem with the outlier day provision to provide added financial risk protection
3. Given the variation in patients' clinical circumstances that may impact evaluation and work-up, patients' geographic locations and the willingness and expertise of the referring physician to be involved in pre-transplant testing, consideration should be given to structuring the reimbursement rate for the evaluation, pre-transplant period, and post-transplant time periods on a percentage discount off billed charges basis.
4. The case rate time period typically includes related donor or autologous harvest, the transplant stay, and a specified number of post-infusion days.

5. Reimbursement for unrelated donor testing and stem cell acquisition may be based on invoice or invoice plus mark-up to cover costs related to administration of the unrelated donor search.
6. The setting in which the HSCT procedure is performed, inpatient or outpatient, can influence reimbursement. Pharmaceuticals may be reimbursed at a higher level per dollar of charge in the outpatient setting. The differences in reimbursement based on setting can have a significant impact on the financial performance of the HSCT program.

2.4 INTEGRATED STRUCTURE FOR CONTRACT MANAGEMENT

The significant complexity of contracting for HSCT services can be demonstrated by the implementation of separate transplant specialty contracting personnel by hospitals and payers. Development of rate structures that support the center's strategic initiatives, monitoring of the center's performance on each contract, and providing assistance to patients in understanding their benefits as they relate to the contract require an integrated team approach.

1. A typical team for contract management would include
   a. Managed care contracting
   b. HSCT program medical director
   c. HSCT program administrator
   d. Patient billing services
   e. Financial counseling personnel
   f. Program's managed care clinical liaison/coordinator:
      i. Review of patient referral insurance information
      ii. Review of patients' benefits
         – Lifetime maximum
         – Transplant maximum
         – Prescription coverage
      iii. Communication with patient regarding benefits
      iv. Liaison with insurance company in communication of patients' status in the process
   g. Medical social worker

2.5 PRIVATE PAYERS

There is significant variability among commercial insurers in all aspects of coverage for HSCT. Private payers often follow

Medicare guidelines for coverage determinations for indications for transplant. Reimbursement structures, benefit packages, donor search and acquisition, financial caps, and clinical trial coverage are examples of areas in which this variation is evident.

1. Centers of Excellence and National Transplant Networks
    a. Many of the large insurance and reinsurance companies have Center of Excellence (COE) or National Transplant Network programs. These programs vary in size depending on the types of transplants, the number of insured lives, and the geographic region covered by those insured lives.
    b. Participation in COE programs and national transplant networks allows a transplant center to have access to a greater number of patients. Patients may be directed to the transplant center because they are a participant in the COE. Participation is based on meeting selection criteria typically based on volumes and outcomes. The selection process typically includes submission of program-specific information and disease-specific outcomes information, as well as an onsite inspection of facilities and review of program standards.
    c. Selection criteria vary among payer networks. In return for a potential increase in patient volumes, transplant centers may agree to package their transplant procedures at rates which cause them to assume some financial risk for above-average costs.

2.6 GOVERNMENTAL PAYERS

1. Medicare DRG Reimbursement
    a. Medicare coverage is limited to items and services that are within the scope of a Medicare benefit category. HSCT is a procedure for which Medicare has developed a National Coverage Determination (NCD). Local Coverage Determinations (LCD) may also apply. These local determinations are developed in the absence of regulation or a national coverage policy. Familiarity with coverage information is of obvious importance and is a critical responsibility of the managed care specialists. The national coverage information is available online from the Medicare Coverage Database (MCD). The NCD for HSCT is in Section 110.81 of this database.

b. Under the Medicare Hospital Acquired Conditions (HAC) initiative, hospitals will be penalized with decreased or no reimbursement for services to Medicare patients if the patient has what is considered a preventable event (e.g., hospital-acquired infection, central line infection, falls resulting in harm). This can be problematic for the HSCT program, given the HSCT patient's proclivity to infection due to immune system compromise. Number of readmissions and time between discharge and readmission are also critically examined.

2. Medicaid

There is wide state-to-state variation in Medicaid coverage for HSCT. There may be limitations based on indication for transplant, maximum allowable inpatient days, and inpatient vs. outpatient service provision. Familiarity with coverage information is of obvious importance and is a critical responsibility of the managed care specialists.

2.7 REGULATORY

1. FACT

   a. The Foundation for the Accreditation of Cellular Therapies (FACT) accreditation is voluntary, but has become an almost necessary qualification for a program to be accepted and competitive. Many insurers, Centers of Excellence programs, and National Transplant Networks include FACT accreditation as a requirement for selection/inclusion.

   b. FACT accreditation addresses clinical care, donor management, cell collection, cell processing, and cell administration.

   c. Accreditation is awarded after successful documentation of compliance with FACT standards. Compliance is judged by evaluation of written documentation and through on-site inspections.

2. CIBMTR

   The Center for International Blood and Marrow Transplant Research (CIBMTR), chosen by Health Resources and Services Administration (HRSA), is the contractor for implementation and ongoing management of the Stem Cell Therapeutic Outcomes Database (SCTOD). As one of four components of the C.W. Bill Young Cell Transplantation Program, the SCTOD provides information about allogeneic blood and marrow transplant outcomes. Submission of patient data to the CIBMTR for the SCTOD is a requirement of all transplant centers that perform allogeneic transplants.

3. FDA

  a. The Food and Drug Administration's (FDA) mission is to protect the public health. In May 2005, the FDA created a registration system for establishments that collect, manipulate, and manufacture cellular therapy products. The registration system was created to establish procedures to prevent the introduction, transmission, and spread of communicable disease by cellular therapy products. HSCT programs are required to register and submit a list of all types of cellular therapy products collected or infused in their institution. The registration must be updated annually.

  b. The FDA requires documentation of complaints that involve distributed cellular therapy products which allegedly involve transmission of a communicable disease to the recipient of the product.

  c. Enforcement of the registration and reporting requirements is accomplished by FDA inspections.

2.8 QUALITY

Assessment of a transplant center's quality is performed internally to evaluate all systems and elements that influence the quality of the HSCT product and service, and performed by external agencies to assess conformance with pre-established specifications or standards.

1. Typical measures of quality – overall mortality and non-relapse mortality – can be difficult to compare between transplant centers due to the potentially significant variability between patient populations managed by individual centers.

  a. Independent bodies such as the University Health Care Consortium attempt to bridge the center-to-center variation by creating assessment tools that normalize the data across centers.

  b. Algorithms for risk assessment based on patient characteristics (co-morbidities) prior to transplant and categorization of disease-related characteristics are used to provide enhanced assurance of valid comparison of outcomes across transplant programs.

c. Standardized determinations of severity of illness (SOI) for the transplant stay are derived from the discharge diagnostic codes. Tools have been generated which use this information to make predictions of expected percentage mortality that can be compared to the observed percentage mortality, with the observed:expected ratio used to comparatively standardize outcomes between centers.

2.9 DATA MANAGEMENT

A transplant program's data management enterprise supports compliance with regulatory standards, internal assessment of quality and quality improvement initiatives, and research development. HSCT programs are expected to contribute data regarding transplant procedures to the NMDP, CIBMTR, or similar data repositories. These data are then available for research purposes on outcomes.

2.10 SUMMARY

The ability to maintain and expand an HSCT program requires the efforts of a specialized business team to develop, implement, and manage contracts; personnel knowledgeable of the most current regulatory standards and data reporting requirements; and a clinical team dedicated to the critical ongoing communication with the referring physician. The partnership between referring physicians and the transplant program is supported by communication related to the pre-transplant workup, the transplant stay, and the requirements of ongoing care post-transplant. This partnership is critical to the promotion of long-term survivorship for the HSCT patient.

2.11 RESOURCES

2.11.1 Websites

Foundation for the Accreditation of Cellular Therapies www.thefactwebsite.org
National Marrow Donor Program www.bethematch.com
Center for International Blood and Marrow Transplant Research www.cibmtr.org
American Society for Blood and Marrow Transplantation www.asbmt.org
European Group for Blood and Marrow Transplantation www.ebmt.org

Stem Cell Therapeutic Outcomes Database http://bloodcell. transplant.hrsa.gov

Blood and Marrow Transplant Clinical Trials Network www.bmtctn.net

Medicare http://www.cms.gov/mcd

Reference

Stranges, E. (Thomson Reuters), Russo, C.A. (Thomson Reuters), Frideman, B. (AHRQ). *Procedures with the Most Rapidly Increasing Hospital Costs, 2004–2007*. HCUP Statistical Brief #82. December 2009. Agency for Healthcare Research and Quality, Rockville, MD. http://www.hcup-us.ahrq.gov/reports/statbriefs/sb82.pdf

CHAPTER 3
Stem Cell Sources

Jose Leis

There are various sources of hematopoietic stem cells (HSC) in use today, including bone marrow, peripheral blood, and umbilical cord blood. HSCs may be obtained from autologous (marrow or PBSC) or allogeneic (HLA-matched related [MRD], HLA-matched unrelated [MUD], mismatched related or unrelated donors, and umbilical cord blood [UCB]) sources. An international inventory of the majority of available adult unrelated donors and cord blood units is maintained by Bone Marrow Donors Worldwide (www.bmdw.org). In 2010, there were an estimated 13–14 million adult donors and 400,000–500,000 cord units available for use in HSCT.

3.1 DONOR SELECTION

1. HLA considerations – critical impact on allogeneic HSCT
   a. Single most important factor in outcome
   b. Low-resolution (antigen equivalent) or high-resolution (allele equivalent) typing done at HLA-A, B, C, DRB1, DQ. (DRB3, 4, 5 and DP typing is also performed, but of uncertain importance)
   c. For marrow, 9/10 match associated with worse overall survival (OS), disease-free survival (DFS), treatment-related mortality (TRM), and acute GVHD
   d. No difference if mismatch in marrow at antigen or allele level except for HLA-C (antigen worse than allele)
   e. 10% lower overall survival with each additional mismatch
   f. For PBSCs, antigen mismatch worse than allele mismatch with increased mortality

R.T. Maziarz, S. Slater (eds.), *Blood and Marrow Transplant Handbook*, DOI 10.1007/978-1-4419-7506-5_3, © Springer Science+Business Media, LLC 2011

g. For PBSCs, a C-antigen mismatch confers increased risk for OS, DFS, TRM, and acute GVHD (grades III–IV)

h. Other donor factors such as age, sex, parity, CMV-status, ABO-matching may have weak effects on outcome

2. Donor Screening

a. To ensure safety for the donor and that administration of the HSC product is safe for the recipient

b. Medical history questionnaire should target risk factors for transmission of genetic or infectious diseases

c. Infectious disease testing includes: HIV 1 and 2, HTLV 1 and 2, hepatitis B and C, CMV, West Nile virus, syphilis, HSV 1 and 2, VZV, and Chagas disease

d. Physical examination, urinalysis, ECG, chest X-ray

e. Baseline laboratory testing: CBC, comprehensive metabolic panel, LDH

3.2 BONE MARROW

1. Gold standard of allogeneic HSCT for three decades

2. Advantages

a. Less T-cells in graft compared with peripheral blood source

b. Decreased risk of chronic GVHD

c. Decreased mortality in children and adolescents

3. Disadvantages

a. Requires operating room, spinal or general anesthesia

b. Increased morbidity to donors

i. Potential risks include pain, infection, blood loss, nerve and musculoskeletal damage

ii. May require blood transfusions for young pediatric donors

c. Slower neutrophil and platelet engraftment

d. Increased risk relapse in some studies

4. Target cell dose

a. Minimum 1×10^8 total mononuclear cells (TMNC)/kg body weight of recipient

b. Target dose 2×10^8 TMNC/kg body weight of recipient

3.3 PERIPHERAL BLOOD (PBSC)

1. Has largely replaced marrow as primary sources of HSCs

a. Principal and preferred source of all autologous HSCT products

    b. Primary source of adult allogeneic HSC

    c. Pediatric allogeneic HSCT – marrow still preferred over PBSC

2. Advantages

    a. Rapid recovery of hematopoiesis compared to marrow

    b. Decreased morbidity to donors

    c. Increased OS and DFS in high-risk hematologic malignancies

3. Disadvantages

    a. Must mobilize stem cells into circulation for peripheral collection

       i. Use of chemotherapy can augment collection in autologous setting

      ii. High-dose G-CSF, GM-CSF, plerixafor are only FDA-approved agents; plerixafor approved for autologous use only

    b. More T-cells in circulation compared with marrow (issue for allogeneic HSCT)

       i. Increased risk of chronic GVHD

4. Target cell dose

    a. Minimum 2×10^6 CD34+ stem cells/kg body weight of recipient

    b. Target 5×10^6 CD34+ stem cells/kg body weight of recipient

    c. Doses $>8 \times 10^6$ CD34+ stem cells/kg are associated with increased risk of GVHD and decreased overall survival in some allogeneic HSCT studies

5. Mobilization

    a. Autologous transplant

       i. Disease-specific chemotherapy followed by high-dose G-CSF 10 µg/kg/day SC until peripheral blood CD34 count increases above institutional target levels, e.g., >10 cells/µl before onset of leukapheresis

      ii. High-dose G-CSF 10 µg/kg/day SC for 4 days followed by leukapheresis on day 5

      iii. High-dose G-CSF 10 µg/kg/day SC for 4 days in the morning + plerixafor 0.24 mg/kg SC (maximum dose 40 mg) on evening day 4

      iv. Plerixafor (Mozobil®)

        – Reversibly inhibits binding of SDF-1α, expressed on bone marrow stromal cells, to the CXC chemokine receptor 4 (CXCR4), resulting in mobilization of hematopoietic stem and progenitor cells from the marrow to the peripheral blood.

- Reduce dose to 0.16 mg/kg (max 27 mg) if estimated GFR < 50 ml/min using Cockroft–Gault equation.
- FDA approval for autologous setting in multiple myeloma and non-Hodgkin lymphoma. Not approved for allogeneic donors.

b. Factors associated with poor mobilization
   i. Prior chemotherapy: increased cycles and duration of treatment
   ii. Prior radiation to marrow
   iii. Low pre-mobilization platelet count
   iv. Female gender
   v. Exposure to purine analogs, e.g., fludarabine
   vi. Exposure to alkylating agents, e.g., prior melphalan in myeloma
   vii. Exposure to lenalidomide
   viii. Marrow involvement by lymphoma
   ix. Low peripheral blood CD34 count during mobilization
   x. Peripheral blood CD34 count has been shown to be proportional to CD34 leukapheresis yield
   xi. Peripheral blood CD34 < 10 cells/μl associated with mobilization failure

c. Strategies for the hard-to-mobilize patient
   i. BID dosing of G-CSF 5–10 μg/kg/day SC for 4 days, then leukapheresis
   ii. Double growth factor: BID dosing of G-CSF 5–10 μg/kg/day SC plus GM-CSF 250 mg/m^2 once daily for 4 days, then leukapheresis
   iii. High-dose G-CSF + plerixafor
   iv. Bone marrow harvest

d. Risk adapted approach: Mayo Clinic
   i. Start G-CSF alone 10 μg/kg/day
   ii. If day 4 or day 5 PB CD34 > 10/μl, initiate leukapheresis the following day
   iii. If day 5 PB CD34 <10/μl, add plerixafor 0.24 mg/kg evening dose, initiate leukapheresis the following morning
   iv. If daily apheresis yield <0.5 × 10^6 CD34/kg, repeat plerixafor and continue leukapheresis the following day
   v. Continue daily G-CSF and plerixafor until goal is reached or STOP if <0.5 × 10^6 CD34/kg collected despite use of plerixafor

3.4 UMBILICAL CORD BLOOD

1. Each year no suitable related or unrelated donor can be identified for 6000–10,000 patients who could potentially benefit from HSCT. This is particularly true for minority patients.
2. Typically, cord blood units typed at intermediate-resolution for HLA-A and HLA-B and at high-resolution for HLA-DR.
3. Advantages
   a. Criteria for a "match" less stringent
      i. 4/6 match acceptable
      ii. Increases chance of finding a suitable donor
   b. UCB lymphocytes are less alloreactive
   c. Allows for greater HLA-disparity, can engraft with 4/6 match
   d. Less GVHD for degree of mismatch
   e. Rapid access: suitable cord unit can be identified in a few days and shipped overnight
4. Disadvantages
   a. Cell dose
      i. Need a minimum of $3–4 \times 10^7$ total nucleated cells (TNC)/kg to ensure durable engraftment
      ii. Only 10% of UCB units have sufficient stem cells to transplant a patient >50 kg in weight
      iii. Increased non-relapse mortality to 70% in $<1.7 \times 10^7$ TNC/kg
   b. Slow engraftment relative to related or unrelated donor marrow or PBSC transplants
   c. Increased infectious complications from slow neutrophil engraftment
   d. No DLI available for treatment of relapse or graft failure
   e. Limited inventory available currently
5. Impact of cell dose
   a. Slow rate of hematopoietic recovery
   b. High risk of graft rejection
   c. High TRM
   d. Poor OS if low dose
   e. Magnified effect of HLA mismatch
6. Choosing the best cord unit (EuroCord recommendations)
   a. 6/6 match $>3 \times 10^7$ TNC/kg
   b. 5/6 match $>4 \times 10^7$ TNC/kg
   c. 4/6 match $>5 \times 10^7$ TNC/kg
   d. Do not perform single-unit UCBT with < 4/6 match or < 3 $\times 10^7$ TNC/kg
7. Strategies to improve UCBT in adults
   a. Double UCB unit grafts to augment cell dose

b. Most patients have more than one 4–6/6 HLA-matched UCB unit available
c. Adults studies suggest improved engraftment and reduced TRM compared with single-unit transplants
d. Sustained engraftment seen from only one of the two units, not both

References

Barker, J. (2007). Umbilical cord blood (UCB) transplantation: An alternative to the use of unrelated volunteer donors? *Hematology Am Soc Hematol Educ Program*, 55–61.

Bensinger, W., Martin, P., Storer, B., Clift, R., Forman, S., Negrin, R., et al. (2001). Transplantation of bone marrow as compared with peripheral blood cells from HLA-identical relatives in patients with hematologic cancers. *N Engl J Med*, 344:175–181.

Confer, D. (February 24, 2010). Traditional perspectives on non-HLA factors in donor search. *Presented in the Selection of Adult Unrelated HSC Donors: Beyond HLA mini-symposium at 2010 BMT Tandem Meetings*. Orlando, Florida.

Eapen, M., Horowitz, M., Klein, J., Champlin, R., Loberiza, F., Ringden, O., et al. (2004). Higher mortality rates after allogeneic peripheral-blood transplatation compared with bone marrow in children and adolescents. *J Clin Oncol*, 22:4872–4880.

Lee, S., Klein, J., Haagenson, M., Baxter-Lowe, L.C., Eapen, M., Fernandez-Vina, M., et al. (2007). High-resolution donor-recipient HLA matching contributes to the success of unrelated donor marrow transplantation. *Blood*, 110:4576–4583.

Micallef, I., Inwards, D., Dispenzieri, A., Gastineua, D., Gertz, M., Hayman, S., et al. (2010). A risk adapted approach utilizing plerixafor in autologous peripheral blood stem cell mobilization. *Biol Blood Marrow Transpl*, 16(1):S197–S198.

Peters, C., Cornish, J., Parikh, S., Kurtzberg, J. (2010). Stem cell source and outcome after hematopoietic stem cell transplantation (HSCT) in children and adolescents with acute leukemia. *Pediatr Clin N Am*, 57:27–46.

CHAPTER 4
Pre-transplant Evaluation

Andy Chen

Conventional hematopoietic stem cell transplant (HSCT) is a vigorous procedure with significant risk for non-infectious and infectious complications. Reduced-intensity HSCT is often offered to recipients with advanced age and/or significant comorbid clinical conditions. Appropriate identification of recipients who will likely have a chance for benefiting from these rigorous procedures is essential. Screening of donors is necessary to identify all potential risks of harm to the donor and to identify potential transmissible illnesses to the recipient.

4.1 CONSIDERATIONS AND/OR INDICATIONS FOR TRANSPLANT

1. Adult acute myelogenous leukemia
   a. Antecedent hematologic disease
   b. Therapy-related AML
   c. Induction failure
   d. CR1 with intermediate- or poor-risk cytogenetics (see Table 4.1)
   e. CR2 and beyond
2. Pediatric acute myelogenous leukemia
   a. High risk (monosomy 5 or 7, age <2 years, induction failure)
   b. CR1 with HLA-matched sibling donor
   c. CR2 and beyond
3. Adult acute lymphoblastic leukemia
   a. CR1 with standard risk up to age 55
   b. CR1 with high risk

R.T. Maziarz, S. Slater (eds.), *Blood and Marrow Transplant Handbook*, DOI 10.1007/978-1-4419-7506-5_4, © Springer Science+Business Media, LLC 2011

TABLE 4.1. Risk stratification for cytogenetics

Risk group	Cytogenetics	Molecular markers
Good	Inv(16); t(16;16) t(8;21) t(15;17)	Normal cytogenetics with isolated NPM1 mutation Normal cytogenetics with isolated CEBPA mutation
Intermediate	Normal +8 only t(9;11) Other abnormalities not defined	Inv(16), t(16;16), and t(8;21) with c-kit mutation
Poor	Complex (≥ 3 abnormalities) −5, del 5q −7, del 7q 3q21q26 t(6;9) t(9;22) 11q23 abnormalities except t(9;11) 17p abnormalities	Normal cytogenetics with Flt3 mutation

      i. BCR-ABL t(9;22)

     ii. MLL (11q23) rearrangements

    iii. High WBC at diagnosis (>30,000 for B cell, >100,000 for T cells)

  c. Induction failure

  d. CR2 and beyond

4. Pediatric acute lymphoblastic leukemia

  a. High risk

      i. Induction failure

     ii. Ph+

    iii. MLL rearrangement

    iv. E2A rearrangement

     v. Burkitts

    vi. Infant

   vii. WBC at diagnosis >100 K

  b. CR1 duration <18 months

  c. CR3 and beyond

5. Myelodysplastic syndrome

  a. INT-1, INT-2, or high-risk IPSS

TABLE 4.2. International prognostic staging system

Prognostic variable	0	0.5	1	1.5	2
Marrow blasts	<5	5–10		11–20	21–30
Karyotype	Good	Intermediate	Poor		
Cytopenias	0–1	2–3			

    b. International Prognostic Staging System (IPSS) (see Table 4.2)
        i. Karyotype
          – Good: normal, −Y only, del(5q) only, del (20q) only
          – Intermediate: +8, single miscellaneous, double miscellaneous
          – Poor: complex (≥3 abnormalities), chromosome 7 abnormality
       ii. Cytopenias
          – Hemoglobin <10 g/dL
          – ANC <1,800 /μL
          – Platelets <100,000 /μL
6. Chronic myelogenous leukemia
    a. No hematologic or minor cytogenetic response within 3 months of frontline therapy
    b. No complete cytogenetic response within 6–12 months of frontline therapy
    c. Disease progression
        i. Demonstrate failure to second-generation tyrosine kinase inhibitor (TKI)
       ii. Development of T3151-resistant mutation
      iii. Progression to accelerated or blast phase of their malignancy
    d. Primary accelerated phase after appropriate disease reduction with TKI therapy (either imatinib or second-generation agent)
    e. Primary blast crisis (myeloid or lymphoid) after appropriate disease reduction with TKI therapy (either imatinib or second-generation agent)
7. Follicular and low-grade non-Hodgkin's lymphoma
    a. relapsed disease, especially second or later
    b. Transformation to DLBCL
8. Diffuse large B-cell lymphoma (see Table 4.3)
    a. Chemosensitive relapse
    b. First line auto HSCT not recommended

TABLE 4.3. International prognostic index (IPI)

Risk factors
Age >60
Performance status >1
Elevated LDH
Extranodal sites >1
Stage III–IV

Risk group	Number of factors
Low	0–1
Low intermediate	2
High intermediate	3
High	4–5

9. Mantle cell NHL
   a. Following initial therapy
10. Hodgkin's lymphoma
    a. No CR with initial therapy
    b. First or subsequent relapse
11. Multiple myeloma
    a. After initiation of therapy (first consolidation)
    b. At progression or relapse
12. Germ cell cancer
    a. Refractory to induction
    b. Second or subsequent relapse
13. Bone marrow failure states
    a. Severe aplastic anemia
    b. Fanconi anemia
    c. Pure red cell aplasia
    d. Amegakaryocytosis
    e. Paroxysmal nocturnal hemoglobinuria
14. Congenital/inherited immune disorders
    a. Severe combined immunodeficiency
    b. Wiskott-Aldrich syndrome
    c. Familial hemophagocytic lymphohistiocytosis
15. Congenital hemoglobinopathies
    a. Beta thalassemia major
    b. Sickle cell disease
16. Congenital metabolic disorders
    a. Hurler's syndrome
    b. Adrenoleukodystrophy
    c. Metachromatic leukodystrophy

4.2 SOURCES OF HEMATOPOIETIC STEM CELLS (SEE TABLE 4.4)

1. Autologous
   a. Peripheral blood
   b. Bone marrow
2. Allogeneic
   a. Related, unrelated
   b. Matched, mismatched, haplo-identical
   c. Peripheral blood, bone marrow, single cord, double cord

TABLE 4.4. Transplant types by disease

Disease	Autologous	Allogeneic
AML	X	X
ALL		X
MDS		X
CML		X
Lymphoma	X	X
Myeloma	X	X
Germ cell	X	
Bone marrow failure		X
Congenital disorders		X

4.3 PATIENT EVALUATION

1. History
   a. Signs/symptoms at diagnosis, pathology, staging, risk stratification, relapses
   b. Treatment history with responses and dates
   c. Complications, both therapy and disease related
   d. Infectious disease history
2. Current disease status
   a. Recent PET and/or CT
   b. Recent bone marrow biopsy
   c. Tumor markers
3. Allergies and medications (including supplements)
4. Past medical history
   a. Chronic or serious illnesses and surgeries
   b. Transfusion history
   c. Vaccinations
   d. Menstrual status (if applicable)
   e. Pregnancies and outcomes

5. Family history
   a. Health status and malignancy history
   b. Potential donors
6. Psycho-social evaluation
   a. Caregiver availability
   b. Psychiatric history
   c. Substance abuse
   d. Work and living situation
   e. Travel history
   f. Financial screening and evaluation
7. Systems evaluation
   a. Dentition
   b. Respiratory including PFTs and DLCO
   c. Cardiac including EKG and ejection fraction (Echo or MUGA)
   d. Hepatic – LFTs
   e. Renal – electrolytes, BUN, creatinine
   f. Neurologic – assess for CNS involvement if indicated
   g. Hematologic – CBC, Blood type (ABO/Rh)
8. Other laboratories/testing
   a. Pathology review
   b. Pregnancy test (if applicable)
   c. Infectious disease testing
      i. Required by Foundation for the Accreditation of Cellular Therapy (FACT):
         – HIV-1 and 2, HepB, HepC, syphilis
      ii. Recommended (required by some authorities):
         – CMV, EBV, HSV, VZV, HTLV-1 and 2, West Nile, Chagas, Toxo
      iii. Selected cases:
         – TB – exposure risk
         – Fungus – past history, allogeneic transplant
         – Parasites – exposure risk, travel history
   d. HLA typing (for Allo candidates)
      i. HLA-A, -B, -DRB1 (also -C if unrelated)
9. Performance status (see Tables 4.5 and 4.6)

4.4 GENERAL GUIDELINES FOR PATIENT ELIGIBILITY
1. Disease meets indication for transplant
2. Chemosensitive disease
   a. Minimal marrow involvement for autologous transplant
      i. Prefer <10% for myeloma; <5% for all others

TABLE 4.5. ECOG performance scale

Score	
0	Fully active, able to carry on all pre-disease performance without restriction
1	Restricted in physically strenuous activity, but ambulatory and able to carry out work of a light or sedentary nature, e.g., light housework, office work
2	Ambulatory and capable of all self-care, but unable to carry out any work activities; up and about more than 50% of waking hours
3	Capable of only limited self-care and confined to bed or chair; more than 50% of waking hours
4	Completely disabled, cannot carry on any self-care; totally confined to bed or chair
5	Dead

TABLE 4.6. Karnofsky performance scale

Score	
100%	Normal, no symptoms or signs of active disease
90%	Able to carry on normal activity, minor signs or symptoms of active disease
80%	Normal activity with effort
70%	Unable to do active work, cares for self
60%	Requires occasional assistance
50%	Requires considerable assistance and frequent medical care
40%	Disabled, needs special care
30%	Hospitalized, death not imminent
20%	Hospitalized, critical condition
10%	Moribund
0	Dead

3. Adequate performance status (see above)
   a. ECOG ≤ 2 or Karnofsky $\geq 70\%$ for conventional ablative regimen
   b. ECOG ≤ 3 or Karnofsky $\geq 50\%$ for reduced intensity transplant
4. Adequate non-hematopoietic organ function
   a. Creatinine $\leq 2\times$ ULN or CrCl ≥ 50 (except amyloid/myeloma)
   b. Cardiac EF $\geq 40\%$, no significant CHF symptoms, no uncontrolled arrhythmia
   c. FEV1, FVC, DLCO $\geq 45\%$ predicted

    d. AST & ALT $\leq 3 \times$ ULN; total bilirubin $\leq 2 \times$ ULN unless Gilbert's syndrome

5. Psycho-social

    a. Ability to provide informed consent
    b. Willing and able to comply with therapy
    c. Available caregiver
    d. Insurance coverage

6. Adequately matched available donor or adequate collection of autologous stem cells

    a. Auto collection: minimum $\geq 2 \times 10^6$ CD34+ cells/kg (ideal $\geq 5 \times 10^6$)
    b. Allogeneic matching
        i. Related: 5–6 of 6 (HLA-A, B, DRB1)
        ii. Unrelated: 7–8 of 8 (HLA-A, B, C, DRB1)
        iii. Cord: 4–6 of 6 (HLA-A, B, DRB1)
        iv. HLA-A mismatch is highest risk
        v. Antigen mismatch is higher risk than allele mismatch
        vi. NMDP does not match for HLA-DRB (3–5) or HLA-DQ

7. No active infections requiring ongoing therapy except

    a. Stable fungal infection on therapy
    b. Prophylactic/suppressive therapy
    c. HIV on HAART

8. Exclusion criteria

    a. Chemo-refractory disease (except selected Hodgkin's)
    b. Life expectancy severely limited by illness other than malignancy
    c. Inability to tolerate cytoreductive chemotherapy
    d. Pregnancy

9. Relative contraindications

    a. Active substance abuse
    b. Lack of insurance/financial resources
    c. Major medical comorbidities
    d. Major psychiatric illness

10. Hematopoietic Cell Transplant Comorbidity Index (see Table 4.7)

    a. Predictor of non-relapse mortality in ablative allogeneic transplants
    b. Consider reduced intensity regimen if comorbidity index ≥ 4

TABLE 4.7. Comorbidity index

Comorbidity	Definition	Points
Arrhythmia	Atrial fibrillation or flutter, sick sinus syndrome, or ventricular arrhythmia	1
Cardiac	Coronary artery disease[a], congestive heart failure, myocardial infarction, or EF $\leq$50%	1
Inflammatory bowel disease	Crohn's disease or ulcerative colitis	1
Diabetes	Requiring treatment with insulin or oral hypoglycemic agents, but not diet alone	1
Cerebrovascular accident	Transient ischemic attack or cerebrovascular accident	1
Psychiatric disturbance	Depression or anxiety requiring psychiatric consult or treatment	1
Hepatic – mild	Chronic hepatitis, bilirubin > ULN – 1.5× ULN, or AST/ALT > ULN – 2.5× ULN	1
Obesity	Body mass index >35 kg/m^2	1
Infection	Requiring continuation of antimicrobial treatment after day 0	1
Rheumatologic	SLE, RA, polymyositis, mixed CTD, polymyalgia rheumatica	2
Peptic ulcer	Requiring treatment	2
Moderate/severe renal	Serum creatinine >2 mg/dL, on dialysis, or prior renal transplantation	2
Moderate Pulmonary	DLCO and/or FEV1 66–80% or dyspnea on slight activity	2
Prior solid tumor	Treated at any time point in patient's past history, excluding non-melanoma skin cancer	3
Heart valve disease	Except mitral valve prolapse	3
Severe Pulmonary	DLCO and/or FEV1 $\leq$65% or dyspnea at rest or requiring oxygen	3
Moderate/severe hepatic	Liver cirrhosis, bilirubin >1.5× ULN or AST/ALT >2.5× ULN	3

[a]One or more vessel-coronary artery stenosis requiring medical treatment, stent, or bypass graft

EF indicates ejection fraction; ULN, upper limit of normal; SLE, systemic lupus erythematosis; RA, rheumatoid arthritis; CTD, connective tissue disease; DLCO, diffusion capacity of carbon monoxide; FEV1, forced expiratory volume in 1 s; AST, aspartate aminotransferase; ALT, alanine aminotransferase

4.5 ALLOGENEIC DONOR EVALUATION

1. HLA typing for HLA-A, -B, -DRB1 (also -C if unrelated)
2. History and physical
3. Transmissible disease screen
   a. Vaccination, travel, transfusion
   b. High-risk history or behaviors
   c. Inherited, hematologic, autoimmune, or malignant conditions
4. Pregnancy history
5. Laboratories
   a. CBC, chemistries, LFTs, coagulation
   b. Blood type and compatibility
   c. Serum pregnancy test (if applicable)
6. Infectious disease
   a. Required by FACT:
      – HIV-1, HIV-2, HepB, HepC, syphilis
   b. Recommended (required by some authorities):
      – CMV, EBV, HSV, HTLV-1, HTLV-2, VZV, West Nile, Chagas
7. Consents and notifications
   a. Donor consent for mobilization therapy and possible line placement
   b. Notify prospective donor of abnormal findings
   c. Document rationale and consent for use of ineligible donor
   d. Notify apheresis unit of health issues that could affect safety of collection

References

FACT -JACIE *International Standards for Cellular Therapy Product Collection, Processing, and Administration.* 4th Ed. (2008).

Greenberg, P., Cox, C., LeBeau, M.M., Fenaux, P., Morel, P., Sanz, G., et al. (1997). International scoring system for evaluating prognosis in myelodysplastic syndromes. *Blood*, 89:2079–2088.

Oliansky, D.M., Gordon, L.I., King, J., Laporl, G., Leonard, J.P., McLaughtin, P., et al. (2010). The role of cytotoxic therapy with hematopoietic stem cell transplantation in the treatment of follicular lymphoma: an evidence-based review. *Biol Blood Marrow Transplant*, 16:443–468.

Oliansky, D.M., Czuczman, M., Fisher, R.I., Irwin, F.D., Lazarus, H.M., Omel, J., et al. (2010). The role of cytotoxic therapy with hematopoietic stem cell transplantation in the treatment of diffuse large B cell lymphoma: update of the 2001 evidence-based review. *Biol Blood Marrow Tansplant*, epub 23 July 2010.

Sorror, M.L., Maris, M.B., Storb, R., Baron, F., Sandmaier, B.M., Malone, D.G., et al. (2005). Hematopoietic cell transplant (HSC)-specific comorbidity index: a new tool for risk assessment before allogeneic HCT. *Blood*, 106:2912–2919.

The International Non-Hodgkin's Lymphoma Prognostic Factors Project. (1993). A predictive model for aggressive non-Hodgkin's lymphoma. *N Eng J Med*, 987–994.

www.asbmt.org/policystat/policy.html

www.marrow.org/physician/tx_indications_timing_referral/index.html

CHAPTER 5
Conditioning Regimens

Joseph Bubalo

The preferred conditioning regimen should be capable of eliminating or reducing the tumor load from the malignant disorder, provide adequate immunosuppression to prevent graft rejection, and have manageable side effects or regimen-related toxicities. Traditionally, all allogeneic conditioning regimens were ablative, meaning that stem cell support was required in order to attain hematopoietic recovery of the bone marrow. More recently, there has been a trend in multiple patient populations to move toward reduced-intensity regimens (RIT), which are defined as any regimen that does not require stem cell support for hematopoietic recovery and results in low hematologic toxicity and mixed donor–recipient chimerism in a substantial proportion of patients in the early post-transplantation period. Most transplantation experts agree that any regimen that includes (i) Total Body Irradiation (TBI) of <500 cGy as a single fraction or <800 cGy if fractionated, (ii) <9 mg/kg of oral busulfan, (iii) <140 mg/m^2 of melphalan, or <10 mg/kg of thiotepa is a RIT regimen.

In the autologous setting, high-dose therapy with stem cell support is frequently done to salvage relapsed or persistent disease as well as to consolidate or prolong cancer remissions. Sequential or tandem stem cell transplants are used in some disease states to further deepen a remission, increase chance for cure, or to facilitate delivery of a high-dose regimen.

R.T. Maziarz, S. Slater (eds.), *Blood and Marrow Transplant Handbook*, DOI 10.1007/978-1-4419-7506-5_5, © Springer Science+Business Media, LLC 2011

.1 COMMON CONVENTIONAL (ABLATIVE) CONDITIONING REGIMENS

Regimen	Disease states treated	Comments
Cy2 or Cy4 + ATG ± TBI	Aplastic anemia	TBI added for unrelated donors (URD)
tBu16Cy2	AML, ALL, CLL, CML, NHL, MM, MDS	
Cy2 – TBI 1200–1400	AML, ALL, CLL, NHL, MDS	
BEAM	NHL, HD, MM	

Cy – cyclophosphamide; ATG – antithymocyte globulin (equine); tBu – targeted busulfan; AML – acute myelogenous leukemia; ALL – acute lymphocytic leukemia; CML – chronic myelogenous leukemia; CLL – chronic lymphocytic leukemia; NHL – non-Hodgkin's lymphoma; HD – Hodgkin's disease; MM – multiple myeloma; MDS – myelodysplasia; BEAM – carmustine, etoposide, cytarabine, melphalan

5.2 COMMON RIT CONDITIONING REGIMENS

Regimen	Disease states treated	Comments
Bu-Flu	AML, ALL, CLL	
Bu-Flu –TBI	AML, ALL, CLL	
Flu-Mel	NHL, MM	
Flu-TBI	AML, ALL, CLL	
TBI – 200 cGY	AML, ALL, CLL	Pace of disease may require more aggressive therapy

Flu – Fludarabine

5.3 COMMON AUTOLOGOUS CONDITIONING REGIMENS

Regimen	Disease states treated	Comments
Bu16-etoposide	AML	
BEAM	NHL, HD	
BuMelTT	NHL, HD	
Carbo-etoposide	Germ cell	May be done in tandem

(Continued)

Regimen	Disease states treated	Comments
Carbo-etoposide-Cy	Germ cell	May be done in tandem
Cy-etoposide-TBI	NHL, HD	
CBV	NHL, HD	
Melphalan	MM, amyloid	May be done in tandem

5.4 CONDITIONING AGENTS

Most conditioning agents are associated with pancytopenia, sterility, and alopecia in the doses used in myeloablative regimens. Mucositis may encompass the entire GI tract and result in stomatitis, esophagitis, nausea, vomiting, and diarrhea. Selected toxicities and points of care are presented, as these are unique or more prevalent in the high-dose therapy setting. On a day-to-day basis, these effects may require additional therapy or attention to care to manage the patient and minimize morbidity.

1. Antithymocytic Immune Globulin (ATG or ATGAM®)
   a. Type: immune modulator, polyclonal MAB
   b. Dose: 30 mg/kg IV daily for 3 days
   c. Toxicities
      i. Fatal allergic reactions. Requires test dose prior to initiation of treatment.
      ii. Serum sickness (or maturation syndrome) symptoms including fever, chills, hypotension, rash, arthralgias, joint pain, and renal insufficiency
   d. Patient care points
      i. Intradermal test dose prior to first dose with contralateral saline dose
      ii. Premed with diphenhydramine, acetaminophen, and steroids
      iii. Run slowly to begin, then may accelerate rate as tolerated
      iv. Have emergency meds (epinephrine, hydrocortisone, diphenhydramine at bedside)
   e. Rabbit ATG (Thymoglobulin®) can be substituted in some circumstances, often based on institutional guidelines
2. Carmustine (BiCNU®, BCNU)
   a. Type: Nitrosourea alkylating agent

  b. Dose: 300 mg/m^2 IV for 1 day and 150 mg/m^2 daily for 3 days are common dose schedules

  c. Toxicities

   i. Infusional hypotension related to rate of administration. See maximum infusion rate.

   ii. Nausea and vomiting

   iii. Progressive pulmonary fibrosis; acute onset usually responds to steroids, but if unresponsive may be fatal. Symptoms include cough, dyspnea or restrictive pattern on PFTs

   iv. Mucositis

  d. Patient care points

   i. Pre-administration baseline PFTs with DLCO

   ii. Administer at a maximum rate of 3 mg/m^2 per minute.

   iii. Requires pre- and post-hydration

3. Busulfan (Myleran®, Busulfex®)

  a. Type: Alkylating agent

  b. Dose (adjusted body weight = IBW + 0.25 (Actual – Ideal Body weight)

   i. Myeloablative = 1 mg/kg/dose PO or 0.8 mg/kg/dose IV every 6 h for total of 12–16 mg/kg

   ii. Reduced intensity = 3.2 mg/kg IV once

   iii. IV dose is 0.8 mg IV per 1 mg PO

  c. Toxicities

   i. Lowers seizure threshold

   ii. Nausea and vomiting

   iii. Pulmonary fibrosis (busulfan lung): symptoms of cough, dyspnea, low-grade fever

   iv. Hepatitis/SOS (may have late onset)

   v. Mucositis

   vi. Hyperpigmentation/skin blistering

  d. Patient care points

   i. Anticonvulsants required to prevent seizures. Loading dose of phenytoin, levetiracetam and/or clonazepam, lorazepam, etc., given the evening prior to first dose of busulfan with maintenance dosing daily continuing through the morning after the administration of the last dose.

   ii. Pharmacokinetic targeting is ideal for oral delivery and can optimize IV administration. Target levels of busulfan (with cyclophosphamide only, not BuMelTT or other busulfan conditioning schedules)

- AUC 950–1,350 μmol minutes for leukemias other than CML or MDS
- AUC 1,315–1,500 μmol minutes for CML
- AUC 1,000–1,350 μmol minutes for NHL
- AUC 1,169–1,315 μmol minutes for MDS

iii. Give oral drug on an empty stomach.

iv. If patient vomits in 30 min or less of drug administration and tablets are visible, count tablets and repeat that number of pills. If unsure, repeat entire dose.

v. If patient vomits within 30–60 min of drug administration and tablets are visible, count tablets and repeat that number of pills. If unsure, repeat one-half the dose.

vi. Tablets should be placed in gelatin capsules for ease of consumption.

vii. If there is more than one episode of emesis requiring redosing, change to IV busulfan.

4. Carboplatin (Paraplatin®)
    a. Type: Alkylating agent
    b. Dose: 600–700 mg/m^2/day IV for 3 days
    c. Toxicities
        i. Irreversible ototoxicity
        ii. Delayed nausea and vomiting
        iii. Renal insufficiency
        iv. Electrolyte disturbance – acidosis, hyponatremia
        v. Neurotoxicity
    d. Patient care points
        i. Maintain adequate hydration
5. Cyclophosphamide (Cytoxan®)
    a. Type: Alkylating agent
    b. Dose: 60 mg/kg/day IV daily for 2 days (based on IBW) incorporated into conventional hematologic malignancy conditioning regimens
        i. Aplastic anemia: 50 mg/kg IV daily for 4 days (based on IBW) is commonly used
    c. Toxicities
        i. Hemorrhagic cystitis
        ii. Cardiomyopathy
        iii. Nausea and vomiting
        iv. Mucositis
        v. SIADH
        vi. Histamine reaction characterized by sinus burning, cough, itchy/watery eyes, chest discomfort/tightness
        vii. Gonadal failure

    d. Patient care points
       i. MUGA or echocardiogram pretreatment with baseline LVEF >45%.
      ii. Adequately hydrate patient for 12 h prior to cyclophosphamide dose with NS. The cyclophosphamide should run concurrently with MESNA to protect bladder. The patient is asked to void every 1–2 h during cyclophosphamide administration. Check for hematuria with each void. If the patient should develop hemorrhagic cystitis, continuous bladder irrigation is indicated.
     iii. Diurese to maintain euvolemia.
     iv. Monitor daily intake/output and weights.
      v. Daily chemistries (Na, K+) during infusion days.
     vi. Infuse slowly if histamine reaction occurs and consider pseudoephedrine PRN.

6. Cytosine Arabinoside (ARA-C, Cytosar-U®)
    a. Type: Antimetabolite
    b. Dose: 400 mg/m^2 IV daily for 4 days
    c. Toxicities
       i. Mucositis
      ii. Cerebellar dysfunction: ataxia, nystagmus, slurred speech
     iii. Chemical conjunctivitis
     iv. Acral erythema
      v. Biliary stasis and elevated LFTs
     vi. Fevers, myalgia, bone pain, chest pain
     vii. Capillary leak syndrome

7. Etoposide (VP-16, Vepesid®)
    a. Type: Plant alkaloid, inhibits topoisomerase II
    b. Dose
       i. With carboplatin: 750 mg/m^2 IV daily for 3 days
      ii. With TBI or busulfan: 30–60 mg/kg IV for 1 day
     iii. With BEAM 2–400 mg/m^2/day IV for 4 days
    c. Selected toxicities
       i. Hypersensitivity, anaphylactic type reaction
      ii. Hypotension, usually an infusional reaction
     iii. Mucositis
     iv. Large volume diarrhea
      v. Elevated LFTs. Evaluate dose for bilirubin >5 mg/dL
     vi. Erythema multiforme, plantar palmar erythemia
     vii. Fever
    viii. Peripheral neuropathy
     ix. Cystitis

 d. Patient care points

  i. Premedicate with steroids and diphenhydramine prior to infusion and repeat 2 h into the infusion

  ii. Fluid bolus with 500–1,000 mL NS for hypotension (SBP <85 mmHg or blood pressure decrease >20 mmHg from baseline) during infusion

  iii. If unresponsive to fluid bolus, stop infusion. May consider restarting at a lower dose after pressure stabilizes with additional steroids, antihistamines, and blood pressure support including dopamine 2–5 mcg/kg/min.

  iv. Maintain adequate hydration pre- and post-infusion and do not give diuretics or antihypertensive medications on days of etoposide administration.

  v. Skin rash may require topical steroid treatment.

8. Fludarabine (Fludara®)

 a. Type: Antimetabolite, purine analog

 b. Dose: 30–40 mg/m^2/day for 3–5 days

 c. Selected toxicities

  i. Rare, severe neurologic toxicity (cortical blindness, coma, death)

  ii. Rare hemolytic anemia

  iii. Combination use with pentostatin has resulted in severe pulmonary toxicity

 d. Patient care points

  i. Profound lymphopenia; prophylaxis and surveillance for opportunistic infections important.

9. Melphalan (Alkeran®)

 a. Type: Alkylating agent

 b. Dose:

  i. Single agent: 100 mg/m^2 IV daily for 2 days (standard) or 200 mg/m^2 × 1 day; can be used at 100 or 140 mg/m^2 in some settings in patients with AL amyloidosis or multiple myeloma

  ii. BEAM: 140 mg/m^2 IV for 1 day

  iii. BuMelTT: 50 mg/m^2 IV daily for 2 days

  iv. Creatinine clearance <10 or dialysis: 70 mg/m^2 IV daily for 2 days (MM or amyloid)

  v. Age >75: 70 mg/m^2 IV daily for 2 days (MM or amyloid)

 c. Selected toxicities

  i. Mucositis

  ii. Hyperpigmentation

  iii. Nausea/vomiting

  iv. Arrhythmias

    d. Patient care points

      i. Give immediately after mixing as half-life is short

      ii. Ask patient to suck on ice chips before, during, and after (at least 30 min) infusion to decrease blood flow to oral mucosa to help prevent mucositis. Cryotherapy has been shown to decrease stomatitis.

10. Thiotepa (Thioplex®)

    a. Type: Alkylating agent

    b. Dose: 250 mg/m^2 IV daily for 2 days with BuMelTT

    c. Selected toxicities

      i. Nausea/vomiting

      ii. CNS changes including decline in mental status

      iii. Hepatic changes including late SOS and elevated LFTs

      iv. Pulmonary toxicity

      v. Headache

      vi. Skin desquamation, especially in intertriginous areas as thiotepa is excreted in sweat.

      vii. Mucositis

    d. Patient care points

      i. Consider having patient shower 2–3 times daily during and for 24 h post high-dose thiotepa administration. Use hydrocortisone cream 0.1% underarms, in groin area or face or triamicinolone cream 0.1% for all other areas for skin desquamation.

      ii. Round dose to nearest 15 mg

11. Total Body Irradiation (TBI)

    a. Dose

      i. Non-ablative transplants: 200–500 cGy in a single dose

      ii. Conventional transplantation: 1,200–1,400 cGy given in divided fractions, dose, number, and delivery per institutional guidelines

      iii. Examples of conventional TBI

        – Low-risk disease: 1,200 cGy divided into eight doses delivered BID over 4 days.

        – High-risk disease: 1,400 cGy divided into eight doses delivered BID over 4 days.

    b. Selected toxicities

      i. Sunburn-like rash, diffuse erythema

      ii. Parotiditis

      iii. Cataracts

      iv. Thyroid dysfunction, usually seen late

      v. Nausea/vomiting

     vi. CNS toxicity, leukoencephalopathy
    vii. Acute pneumonitis/alveolar hemorrhage
  viii. Fatigue
     ix. Growth failure
      x. Gonadal failure
     xi. Diarrhea
  c. Patient care points
      i. Premed before each treatment
     ii. Shield lungs as per protocol
   iii. Pretreatment TSH

5.5 ANTIEMETIC DOSING

Agent	Risk	Antiemetic regimen	Comments
Antithy-mocyte globulin	Low	None needed	Other premedications required
Busulfan	Moderate to high	Ondansetron 8 mg PO q 6 h or 24 mg PO daily	Dexamethasone 20 mg daily with once daily ondansetron
Carboplatin	High	Ondansetron 24 mg PO or 8 mg IV prior to first daily chemotherapy dose	Dexamethasone 20 mg daily with each daily ondansetron
Carmustine	High	Ondansetron 24 mg PO or 8 mg IV prior to first daily chemotherapy dose	Dexamethasone 20 mg daily with each daily ondansetron. Would give lorazepam 1 mg to all patients
Cyclophos-phamide	High	Ondansetron 24 mg PO or 8 mg IV prior to first daily chemotherapy dose	Dexamethasone 20 mg daily with each daily ondansetron
Cytarabine	Low (<1000 mg/m^2/day)	Ondansetron 8 mg PO daily. 16 mg (8 mg IV) if other chemotherapy agents given	Dexamethasone 8–12 mg daily with each daily ondansetron

(Continued)

Agent	Risk	Antiemetic regimen	Comments
Etoposide	Moderate to high	Ondansetron 24 mg PO or 8 mg IV prior to first daily chemotherapy dose	Dexamethasone 20 mg daily with each daily ondansetron
Melphalan	High	Ondansetron 24 mg PO or 8 mg IV prior to first daily chemotherapy dose	Dexamethasone 20 mg daily with each daily ondansetron
Total body irradiation	High	Ondansetron 8 mg PO prior to each radiation fraction	Dexamethasone 20 mg daily with the first daily ondansetron
Thiotepa	High	Ondansetron 24 mg PO or 8 mg IV prior to first daily chemotherapy dose	Dexamethasone 20 mg daily with each daily ondansetron

Notes

1. Ondansetron interchangeable with granisetron at equivalent doses. Palonosetron and dolasetron dosing for optimal effect unclear.

2. Lorazepam 0.5–1 mg PO prior to each day's first chemotherapy dose also recommended for most patients.

References

Champlin, R., Khouri, I., Anderlini, P., De Lima, M., Hosing, C., McMannis, J., et al. (2003). Nonmyeloablative preparative regimens for allogeneic hematopoietic transplantation: Biology and current indications. *Oncology*, 17:94–100.

Chunduri, S., Dobogai, L.C., Peace, D., Saunthararajah, Y., Chen, H.Y., Mahmud, N., et al. (2006). Comparable kinetics of myeloablation between fludarabine/full-dose busulfan and fludarabine/melphalan conditioning regimens in allogeneic peripheral blood stem cell transplantation. *Bone Marrow Transplant*, 38:477–482.

Ciurea, S.O., Anderssen, B.S. (2009). Busulfan in hematopoietic stem cell transplantation. *Biol Blood Marrow Transplant*, 15:523–536.

Giralt, S., Ballen, K., Rizzo, D., Bacigalupo, A., Horowitz, M., Pasquini, M., et al. (2009). Reduced intensity conditioning regimen workshop: defining the dose spectrum. Report of a workshop convened by the Center for International Blood and Marrow Transplant Research. *Biol Blood Marrow Transplant*, 15:367–369.

Al-Ali, H., Cross, M., Lange, T., Freund, M., Dolken, G., Niederwieser, D., et al. (2009). Low-dose total body irradiation-based regimens as preparative regimens for allogeneic haematopoietic cell transplantation in acute myelogenous leukemia. *Curr Opin Oncol*, 21(Suppl 1), S17–S22.

Khouri, I. (2006). Reduced-intensity regimens in allogeneic stem-cell transplantation for non-Hodgkins lymphoma and chronic lymphocytic leukemia. *Hematology Am Soc Hematol Educ Program*, 390–397

Lekakis, L., de Padua Silva, L., de Lima, M. (2008). Novel preparative regimens in hematopoietic stem cell transplantation. *Curr Pharm Design*, 14:1923–1935.

Margolin, K., Synold, T., Longmate, J., Doroshow, J.H. (2001). Methodologic guidelines for the design of high dose chemotherapy regimens. *Biol Blood Marrow Transplant*, 7:414–432.

CHAPTER 6
Supportive Care

Bryon Allen

Improved supportive care measures have allowed patients to better tolerate chemoradiotherapy conditioning regimens. The resulting outcomes have improved patients' ability to perform daily activities, maintain oral nutrition, maintain fluid and electrolyte balance, and contribute to decreased treatment-related morbidity. Improved management of pain, diarrhea, nausea, and vomiting has contributed to the evolution of the outpatient hematopoietic stem cell transplant (HSCT) procedure.

6.1 PAIN MANAGEMENT

1. For HSCT patients with new-onset symptoms of pain, utilize oral narcotics early to establish confidence that pain control will be accomplished during the transplant course. Oxycodone (oral), morphine (oral; parenteral), or hydromorphone (oral; parenteral) can be effective in these settings.
2. For patients requiring opioids around the clock to maintain pain control, consider changing to a long-acting oral opioid (MS Contin, Oxycontin) or a patient-controlled analgesia (PCA) basal rate with prn medications for breakthrough pain for most effective analgesia.
   a. Calculate the starting basal dose in non-opioid-naive patients by multiplying the total previous 24-h usage by 0.8 to represent 80% of the patient's baseline chronic pain requirements. Then, divide by 24 to obtain the starting continuous infusion dosage.
   b. For opioid-naive patients, see Table 6.1 for dosing recommendations.

R.T. Maziarz, S. Slater (eds.), *Blood and Marrow Transplant Handbook*, DOI 10.1007/978-1-4419-7506-5_6, © Springer Science+Business Media, LLC 2011

TABLE 6.1. PCA starting dose in opioid-naive patients

Opioid	Demand dose	Lockout (min)	Continuous basal
Morphine	1–2 mg	6–10	0–2 mg/h
Hydromorphone	0.2–0.4 mg	6–10	0–0.4 mg/h
Fentanyl	20–50 mcg	6–10	0–60 mgc/h

Used with permission of Wolters Kluwer Health. Grass (2005)

    c. Increases to basal rate should be based on previous 24-h dosing.

3. Pain should be assessed every 4 h and more frequently as needed to assess the efficacy of analgesic regimen.
   a. A numeric rating scale or similar for adults
   b. The Wong-Baker Faces Pain Scale is recommended for children aged 3 years and younger (Fig. 6.1)

4. For patients with acute kidney injury (serum creatinine >2 mg/dL), fentanyl or hydromorphone is preferred as morphine has active metabolites that can accumulate.

5. Maximize oral symptom relief for patients with mucositis with frequent normal saline rinses and topical analgesics such as "Special Mouthwash" or "Miracle Mouthwash" (1:1:1 mixture of viscous lidocaine/diphenhydramine/aluminum + magnesium hydroxide).

6. Be aware of medications that may potentiate the sedative effects of opioids (benzodiazepines, antihistamines, etc.) and adjust medications appropriately

7. Initiate bowel laxative regimen when patients are receiving ongoing opioid therapy or beginning a PCA. The goal is for the patient to have a bowel movement every 24–48 h without straining. Bowel regimen should be held for loose stools.
   a. Docusate + Senna 50/8.6 mg (Senokot-S®) one to two tablets PO daily to BID
   b. Lactulose 30 mL PO BID
   c. Polyethylene glycol (MiraLax®) 17 g in 4–8 oz fluid daily

8. When patient no longer requires PCA, begin to taper. Consider
   a. Rate of taper is dependent on the length of time patient has been receiving PCA
      i. If ≥7 days, taper hourly rate by 10% of pre-taper dose every 12 h

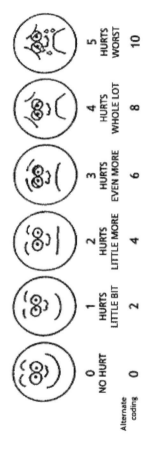

Ask the patient to choose the face that best describes how they are feeling.

FIG. 6.1. **Wong-Baker faces pain scale:** ask the patient to choose the face that best describes how they are feeling. From Hockenberry and Wilson (2009). Used with permission. Copyright Mosby

    ii. If <7 days, taper hourly rate by 10% of pre-taper dose every 8 h

  b. Continue taper as above if pain is tolerable or decreases, or patient does not have signs of withdrawal

  c. Hold taper and adjust opioids as needed if pain is not tolerable or pain increases

  d. Anticipate ongoing need for oral narcotics as substitute, after PCA taper is achieved

  e. If patient shows signs of withdrawal
    i. Consider administration of a bolus of the opioid at 50% of the current hourly rate
    ii. Repeat bolus every 2–4 h until the next dose adjustment is due
    iii. Consider non-pharmacologic interventions and adjuvant drugs
    iv. If withdrawal symptoms have resolved by the time of the next scheduled adjustment, continue taper
    v. If withdrawal symptoms have not resolved, repeat 50% bolus every 2–4 h until the next dose adjustment is due and decrease taper intervals to 10% of pre-taper dosing every 24 h

  f. When the hourly rate of morphine 0.5 mg, hydromorphone 0.1 mg, or fentanyl 5 mcg is reached, maintain that rate for 24 h, then discontinue infusion

  g. If the patient exhibits withdrawal symptoms after discontinuation of the opioid, give a bolus of morphine 0.5 mg, hydromorphone 0.1 mg, or fentanyl 5 mcg (use the same opioid as infusion) every 3–4 h prn. Assess need for prn medications to manage withdrawal symptoms

6.2 NAUSEA

1. Patients with persistent nausea despite prn antiemetics should receive scheduled antiemetics.
  a. Schedule a dopamine antagonist + a short-acting benzodiazepine, e.g. lorazepam (Ativan®) and/or diphenhydramine (Benadryl®).
  b. Lorazepam should not be used alone as a scheduled antiemetic unless for anticipatory nausea.
  c. Examples of dopamine antagonists include:
    i. Prochlorperazine (Compazine®) 5–10 mg PO/IV q 6 h
    ii. Metoclopramide (Reglan®) 20–30 mg PO/IV qAC and HS

    iii. Droperidol (Inapsine®) 0.625 mg IV q 6 h
    iv. Haloperidol (Haldol®) 0.5–2 mg PO/IV q 4–6 h
    v. Promethazine (Phenergan®) 12.5 mg PO/IV q 4–6 h

2. Motion-induced nausea should be treated with either a scopalomine patch (Transderm Scop®) 1.5 mg, changed every 3 days or meclizine (Bonine®, Antivert®) 12.5–15 mg po q 8 h.

3. Serotonin 5-HT3 inhibitors (ondansetron [Zofran®], granisetron [Kytril®]) should not be used as prn agents, nor should they be used post-completion of the conditioning regimen for breakthrough nausea.
    i. These medications have been proven effective for acute nausea, however, not in the setting of delayed nausea.

4. Anticipatory nausea should be treated with lorazepam (Ativan®) or alprazolam (Xanax®) prior to the aggravating factor (e.g., medications, meals).

6.3 DIARRHEA (SEE TABLE 6.2)

1. Patients with frequent loose or watery stools should have stool specimens sent for evaluation for *Clostridium difficile* overgrowth.

2. Once *C. diff* has been ruled out, begin scheduled antidiarrheals
    i. If stool volume ≤1 L/day, begin loperamide (Imodium®) 4 mg po q 6 h.

TABLE 6.2. Diarrhea associated with chemotherapy (not graft-versus-host disease)

Grade	Diarrhea
1	Increase of <4 stools per day over baseline; mild increase in ostomy output compared to baseline
2	Increase of 4–6 stools per day over baseline; IV fluid indicated <24 h; moderate increase in ostomy output compared to baseline; not interfering with ADL
3	Increase of ≥7 stools per day over baseline; incontinence; IV fluids ≥24 h; severe increase in ostomy output compared to baseline; interfering with ADLs
4	Life-threatening consequences (i.e., hemodynamic collapse)
5	Death

    ii. If stool volume >1 L/day or patient has had no response to lower dose, begin/increase loperamide to 4 mg po q 4 h.

    iii. If patient has not had a response to loperamide after 48 h, consider beginning octreotide (Sandostatin®) 250–500 mg IV q 8 h or 100–150 mg SQ TID.

3. Reduce lactose-containing products.
4. Consider changing patient to NPO status to determine if diarrhea is secretory.
5. Consider GI consult for evaluation and management recommendations.

6.4 MUCOSITIS (SEE TABLE 6.3)

1. Normal saline oral rinses can be used every 1–2 h while awake to assist in gentle oral debridement

TABLE 6.3. World Health Organization (WHO) oral mucositis grading scale

Grade 0	No changes
Grade 1	Oral soreness ± erythema. No ulceration
Grade 2	Oral erythema and ulcers; patient able to swallow a solid diet
Grade 3	Oral ulcers; only liquid diet possible
Grade 4	Oral alimentation is not possible

Used with permission of World Health Organization (1979)

2. Discourage the use of dentures, especially at night, once chemotherapy is initiated and particularly in the setting of oral ulceration
3. Once platelet count falls below 50,000/mm^3, discard toothbrush and use sponge toothettes until platelet count recovers to >50,000/mm^3
4. "Special Mouthwash/Miracle Mouthwash" for topical analgesia (see point 5 in Section 6.1)
5. Parenteral pain medication should be encouraged as needed
6. Choose a mechanical soft, non-acidic, and minimally spiced diet

6.5 ACID SUPPRESSION

1. For persistent gastric esophageal reflux disease/gastritis, all patients should receive a proton pump inhibitor, the choice of which depends on institutional formulary.
   a. Lansoprazole (Prevacid®) 30 mg po daily or BID
   b. Omeprazole (Prilosec®) 20 mg po daily or BID
   c. Esomeprazole (Nexium®) 40 mg po daily
   d. Pantoprazole (Protonix®) 40 mg po daily
2. For patients unable to tolerate oral medication or for patients receiving total parenteral nutrition (TPN), substitute famotidine (Pepcid®) 40 mg IV daily. May add to TPN if institutional policy allows.
3. Note: Avoid the use of PPIs and H2 blockers concomitantly with posaconazole (Noxifil®) to avoid decreased absorption of the azole.

6.6 CONSTIPATION

1. If patient has not had a bowel movement in 48 h, begin scheduled senna 8.6 mg (Senokot®) two tablets po qhs. Titrate to maintain an adequate bowel routine for the patient, up to 70–100 mg of senna daily in divided doses.
2. If senna is ineffective to maintain bowel regimen, consider additional agents:
   a. Lactulose 30 mL po q 4 h until BM
   b. Polyethylene glycol (MiraLax®) 17 g in 4–8 oz fluid daily until BM
   c. Magnesium Citrate (Citroma®) 150–300 mL po daily until BM
3. Avoid enemas or suppositories in patients with neutropenia (ANC <1,500/μL) or anticipated neutropenia due to increased risk of infection.

6.7 MENSES

In conditions where bleeding diathesis is predictable (such as in menstruating females undergoing high-dose chemotherapy with resultant thrombocytopenia), pretreatment to induce amenorrhea is indicated. The choice of hormonal therapy is made based on the individual patient and risk of hepatic injury with transaminase elevation. Estrogens are felt to be contraindicated in patients with a history of breast cancer, and can cause transaminitis and bilirubin elevation with resultant confusion regarding the etiology in the setting of transplant-induced hepatic toxicity (i.e., GvHD, sinusoidal obstructive syndrome). Oral agents of any kind may be less effective due to decreased absorption and difficulty of administration due to mucositis or nausea. Intramuscular injections are contraindicated in the presence of significant thrombocytopenia.

1. Hormone therapy should be initiated on admission and discontinued after the female patient has achieved a transfusion-independent platelet count of >50,000/mm^3. If the patient is receiving high-dose oral contraceptives (ethinyl estradiol with progesterone agent/medroxyprogesterone), be certain to reduce to standard dosing once hematologic indices normalize. Additionally, consider alternative pregnancy prevention if hormones are discontinued.
2. Agents that may be used to induce amenorrhea with "hormone neutral" malignancies include:
   a. Medroxyprogesterone (Provera®) 10 mg po daily beginning at the start of conditioning. If no response is obtained in 2–3 days, this may be increased by 10 mg po daily every 2–3 days to a maximum of 30 mg po daily.
      i. If this is unsuccessful in suppression breakthrough bleeding, add ethinyl estradiol/norgestrel (Lo-ovral®) 3 tablets po daily × 3 days, then 2 tablets po daily × 2 days, then 1 tablet po daily (do not take sugar pills).
   b. Medroxyprogesterone (Depo-Provera®) 150 mg IM as one dose given 1 month prior to initiation of high-dose chemotherapy if platelet count is >50,000/mm^3.
   c. Leuprolide acetate (Lupron®) 3.75–7.5 mg IM
      i. See Table 6.4 for dosing schedule
      ii. If drug administration is required during the thrombocytopenic period, dose 1 mg/day SQ until platelet count is >50,000/mm^3.
   d. If patients are unable to tolerate oral medications, the ethinyl estradiol/norelgestromin (Ortho-Evra®) patch can be substituted. This patch should be changed weekly and may be increased to two patches after 3–4 days if additional control is needed.

TABLE 6.4. Schedule of lupron dosing

First injection	Day-37–28
Second injection	Day-7
Third injection	Day+21 if platelets >50,000/mm^3

e. Consider platelet transfusion with increased platelet threshold.
3. If the above measures are inadequate to control vaginal bleeding, a GYN consult should be obtained to investigate alternative etiologies.

6.8 TREMOR

1. For tremors associated with transplant (e.g., calcineurin inhibitors, chronic GvHD), consider propranolol (Inderol®) 10 mg po QID. May increase to 20 mg po QID if no response; however, total daily dose should not exceed 120–320 mg po daily in divided doses.
2. May substitute propranolol LA (Inderal LA®) 60–120 mg po daily for patient convenience.
3. Gabapentin (Neurontin®) 400 mg po TID. Recommend titrating up to total daily dose (400 mg po daily on day 1, 400 mg po BID on day 2, then 400 mg po TID)

References

Aapro, M., Moassiotis, A., Olver, I. (2005). Anticipatory nausea and vomiting. *Support Care Cancer*, 13(2):117–121.

Alffenaar, J.W., VanAssen, S., VanderWerf, T., Kosterink, J.G., Uges, D.R. (2009). Correspondence (Omeprazole significantly reduces posaconazole serum trough level). *CID*, 48(6):2990.

Amsterdam, A., Jakubowiski, A., Castro-Malaspina, H., Baxi, E., Kauff, N., Krychman, M., et al. (2004). Management of menorrhagia. Treatment of menorrhagia in women undergoing hematopoietic stem cell transplantation. *Bone Marrow Transplant*, 34(4):363–366.

Anand, A., Glatt, A. (1993). Clostridium difficile infection associated with antineoplastic chemotherapy. *Clin Infect Dis*, 17(1):109–113.

Barbounis, V., Koumakis, G., Vassilomanolakis, M., Demiri, M., Efremidis, A. (2001). Control of irinotecan-induced diarrhea by octreotide after loperamide failure. *Support Care Cancer*, 9(4): 258–260.

Benson III, A., Catalano, R.B., Engelking, C., Kornblau, S., Matenson Jr, J., McCallum, R., et al. (2004). Recommended guidelines for the treatment of cancer treatment induced diarrhea. *J Clin Oncol*, 22(14):2918–2926.

Davis, M., Weissman, D., Arnold, R. (2004). Opioid dose titration for severe cancer pain: a systematic evidence-based review. *J Palliat Med*, 7(3):462–468.

Dodd, M., Dibble, S., Miakowski, C., MacPhail, L., Greenspan, D., Paul, S., et al. (2000). Randomized clinical trial of the effectiveness of 3 commonly used mouthwashes to treat chemotherapy-induced mucositis. *Oral Surg Oral Med Oral Pathol Oral Radiol Endod,* 90(1):39–47.

Dunbar, P., Buckley, P., Gavrin, J.R., Sanders, J.E., Chapman, C.R. (1995). Use of patient controlled analgesia for pain control for children receiving bone marrow transplant. *J Pain Symptom Manage,* 10(8):604–611.

Epstein, J., Schubert, M. (2004). Managing pain in mucositis. *Semin Oncol Nurs,* 20(1):30–37.

Gates, R., Fink, R. (2008). *Oncology Nursing Secrets.* St. Louis, Missouri, Mosby.

Gibson, R., Keeft, D. (2006). Cancer chemotherapy-induced diarrhea and constipation: mechanisms of damage and prevention strategies. *Support Care Cancer,* 14(9):890–900.

Gironell, A., Kulisevsky, J., Barbanoi, M., Lopez-Villegas, D., Hemandez, G., Pascual-Sedano, B. (1999). A randomized placebo-controlled comparative trial of gabapentin and propranolol in Eesential tremor. *Arch Neurol,* 56(4):475–480.

Grass, J. (2005). Patient-controlled analgesia. *Anesth Analg,* 101(55):S44–S61.

Hockenberry, M.J., Wilson, D. (2009) *Wong's Essentials of Pediatric Nursing,* 8th ed., St. Louis, Missouri, Mosby.

Keefe, D.M., Schubert, M.M., Elting, L.S., Sonis, S.T., Epstein, J.B., Raber-Durlacher, J.E., et al. (2007, February 5). *Updated Clinical Practice Guidelines for the Prevention and Treatment of Mucositis.* Retrieved February 2, 2010, from Wiley InterScience: http://www3.interscience.wiley.com/cgi-bin/fulltext/114078093/PDFSTART

Kovac, A. (2000). Prevention and treatment of postoperative nausea and vomiting. *Drugs,* 59(2):213–243.

Krishna, G., Moton, A., Ma, L., Medlock, M., McLeod, J. (2009). Pharmacokinetics and absorption of posaconazole oral suspension under various gastric conditions in healthy volunteers. *Antimicrob Agents Chemother,* 53(3):958–966.

Lehmann, K. (2005). Recent developments in patient-controlled analgesia. *J Pain Symptom Manage,* 29(5):S72–S89.

Levens, E., Scheinberg, P., DcCherney, A. (2007). Severe menorrhagia associated with thrombocytopenia. *Obstet Gynecol,* 110(4):913–917.

Lexi-Comp, I. (2010, February 2). Lexi-Drugs. http://lexi.com © 2010.

Martin-Johnston, M., Okoji, O., Armstrong, A. (2008). Therapeutic amenorrhea in patients at risk of thrombocytopenia. *Obstet Gynecol Surv,* 63(6):395–402.

Muehlbauer, P.M., Thorpe, D., Davis, A., Drabot, R., Rawlings, B.L., Kiker, E. (2009). Putting evidence into practice: evidence-based interventinos to prevent, manage, and treat chemotherapy-and radiotherapy-induced diarrhea. *Clin J Oncol Nurs,* 13(3):336–342.

National Comprehensive Cancer Network Clinical Practice Guidelines in Oncology[TM]. (n.d.). *Antiemesis.* Retrieved February 2,

2010, from http://www.nccn.org/professinoals/physician_gls/f_guidelines.asp

National Comprehensive Cancer Network Clinical Practice Guidelines in Oncology^{TM}. (n.d.). *Adult Cancer Pain.* Retrieved February 2, 2010, from http://www.nccn.org/professionals/physician_gls/f_guidelines.asp

Nelson, K., Walsh, D., Sheehan, F. (2002). Cancer and chemotherapy-related upper gastrointestinal symptoms: the role of abnormal gastric motor function and its evaluation in cancer patients. *Support Care Cancer*, 10(6):455–461.

Oncology Nursing Society. (2008). *Putting Evidence into Practice: Prevention of Bleeding.* Retrieved February 2, 2010, from http://www.ons.org/Research/PEP/media/ons/docs/research/outcomes/bleeding/tabl-of-evidence.pdf

Parran, C., Pederson, C. (2000). Development of an opioid-taper algorithm for hematopoietic cell transplant recipients. *Oncol Nurs Forum*, 27(6):967–974.

Quaas, A., Ginsburg, E. (2007). Prevention and treatment of uterine bleeding in hematologic malignancy. *Eur J Obstet Gynecol Reprod Biol*, 134(1):3–8.

Raber-Durlacher, J. (1999). Current practices for management of oral mucositis in cancer patients. *Support Care Cancer*, 7, 71–74.

Rapp, S., Ready, L.B., Nessly, M. (1995). Acute pain management in patients with prior opioid consumption: a case-controlled retrospective review. *Pain*, 61(2):195–201.

Smith, S. (2001). Evidence-based management of constipation in the oncology patient. *Eur J Cancer Care*, 5(1):18–25.

Tramonte, S., Brand, M.B., Mulrow, C.D., Amato, M.G., O'Keefe, M.E., Ramirez, G. (1997). The treatment of chronic constipation in adults. *J Ge Intern Med*, 12(1):15–24.

Williamson, A., Hoggart, B. (2005). Pain: a review of three commonly used pain rating scales. *J Clin Nurs*, 14(7):798–804.

Wolfe, M.M., Sachs, G. (2000). Acid suppression: optimizing therapy for gastroduodenal ulcer healing gastric reflux disease, and stress-related erosive syndrome. *Gastroenterology*, 118(2):S9–S31.

Wood, A. (Ed.). (2002). Analgesics for the treatment of pain in children. *N Eng J Med*, 347(14):1094–1102.

World Health Organization. (1979). *Handbook for reporting results of cancer treatment.* Retrieved February 28, 2010, from Geneva: World Health Organization: http://whqlibdoc.who.int/publications/9241700483.pdf

Zesiewicz, T.A., Elble, R., Louis, E.D., Hauser, R.A., Sullivan, K.L., Dewey, J.R., et al. (2005). Practice parameter: therapies for essential tremor. *Neurology*, 64(12):2008–2020.

Zidan, J., Haim, N., Beny, A., Stein, M., Gez, E., Kuten, A. (2001). Octreotide in the treatment of severe chemotherapy-induced nausea. *Ann Oncol*, 12(2):227–229.

CHAPTER 7
Nutrition

Stacey Evert

Hematopoietic stem cell transplant (HSCT) patients have huge metabolic demands related to wound healing after conditioning regimens and infectious events with associated febrile states. In allogeneic transplant patients, the systemic inflammatory state, and local tissue damage imposed by acute graft versus host disease. In the long term, ongoing inflammatory conditions and maldigestion/malabsorption can contribute to a chronic wasting syndrome. The central and critical importance of maintaining adequate nutritional balance throughout the transplant process cannot be understated. Understanding the anabolic and catabolic states seen in the HSCT population, as well as issues related to the restriction of diet for these patients, is essential. While we seek to optimize the nutritional state of the patient, it is also important to recognize that the GI tract can be a portal of infection. As such, the identification of an appropriate diet that limits further infectious risk in this immune-compromised patient population is essential. Within this section, the rationale for a controlled low-bacteria diet is provided with general guidelines. Additionally, details regarding the goals for nutrition during HSCT and guidelines for initiation of total parenteral nutrition (TPN) are given with additional recommendations including a discussion of the ongoing debate regarding L-glutamine, what it is, its uses, and the controversy of its benefit.

7.1 LOW-BACTERIA DIET
Patients undergoing intensive preparative treatment for HSCT who develop a period of cytopenia have an increased risk

R.T. Maziarz, S. Slater (eds.), *Blood and Marrow Transplant Handbook*, DOI 10.1007/978-1-4419-7506-5_7,
© Springer Science+Business Media, LLC 2011

for developing a food-related infection from bacteria, yeasts, molds, viruses, and parasites. To help prevent any food-related infections, many institutions have implemented some form of low-bacteria or low-microbial diet. While the effect of a low-bacteria diet on preventing infection is unknown and more studies are needed to determine the effectiveness, HSCT patients who are neutropenic should avoid foods associated with increased infection risk. The Center for Disease Control (CDC) has developed a list of foods that a HSCT patient should avoid as well as food safety guidelines to follow. These guidelines should be the building block individual institutions use to develop their own version of a low-bacteria diet.

CDC guidelines include the use of separate cutting boards for raw meats and vegetables, care givers thoroughly washing hands after handling raw meats, and cooking meats to the appropriate internal temperature for that product. Foods patients should avoid include:

1. Raw and undercooked eggs and foods containing them
2. Unpasteurized dairy products
3. Unpasteurized fruit and vegetable juices
4. Unpasteurized cheeses or cheeses containing molds
5. Undercooked or raw poultry, meats, fish, and seafood
6. Vegetable sprouts (e.g., alfalfa, bean, and other seed sprouts)
7. Raw fruits with a rough texture (e.g., raspberries)
8. Smooth raw fruits (unless washed under running water, peeled, or cooked)
9. Unwashed raw vegetables (unless washed under running water, peeled, or cooked)
10. Undercooked or raw tofu
11. Raw or unpasteurized honey
12. Deli meats, hot dogs, and processed meats
13. Raw, uncooked grain products
14. Mate tea
15. All moldy and outdated food products
16. Unpasteurized beer
17. Raw, uncooked brewer's yeast
18. Unroasted raw nuts
19. Roasted nuts in the shell

In general, some version of a low-bacteria diet should be followed for 2–3 months post-autologous transplant; allogeneic patients should continue until day +100. In the end, it is up to the patient's provider to determine when the patient can stop following this diet.

Water safety is also a concern for these patients. HSCT patients should avoid using well water as water testing is performed too infrequently. If patients choose to use tap water, they should pay close attention to water advisories and follow them. Use of a water filter or home distiller can reduce the risk for waterborne pathogens that may be found in tap water. The filter "should be capable of removing particles ≥ 1 μm in diameter or filter by reverse osmosis." Bottled water should be used with caution and checked to be sure that either reverse osmosis, distillation, or 1 μm particulate absolute filtration is used to remove Cryptosporidium (patients may need to check with bottler to see if this has been done). Also patients should be aware that the water used to make ice, ice tea, coffee, etc. must be free of Cryptosporidium (this is especially important if patients are not at their own residence).

7.2 GOALS OF NUTRITION DURING TRANSPLANT

Because HSCT patients are predisposed to malnutrition related to the disease process and conditioning regimen toxicities, they should receive ongoing nutrition assessment throughout the transplant process. This includes nutritional and medical histories, anthropometry, chemistry review and assessment of other factors that may interfere with the patient taking adequate nutrition (pain control, activity level, etc.). Using these factors will assist in determining the nutrient requirement for individual patients.

In general, patients who are in the immediate post-transplant phase have the following energy and protein requirements:

1. Energy needs (BEE = Basal Energy Expenditure)
   a. Calculated by Harris Benedict Equations
      i. For men, the BEE = 66.5 + (13.75 × kg) + (5.0 × cm) – (6.78 × age)
      ii. For women, the BEE = 65.1 × (9.56 × kg) + (1.85 × cm) – (4.68 × age)
   b. Baseline needs: BEE × 1.3–1.4 (30–35 kcal/kg, ASPEN Core Curriculum)
      i. Typically used with patients with evidence of engraftment and no metabolic stressors

   c. Stressed needs: BEE × 1.5–1.6
      i. Typically used in the immediate post-transplant period.
2. Protein needs
   a. Estimated as approximately two times the Recommended Dietary Allowance.
   b. 1.5 g/kg – use adjusted weight for obesity: [ideal weight + 0.025 (actual weight – ideal weight)]
   c. Protein requirements may need to be adjusted due to other medical conditions
      i. Increase requirements due to muscle wasting, GHVD, etc.
      ii. Decrease requirements due to renal insufficiency, hepatic encephalopathy, etc.
3. Fluid needs
   a. Should be individualized based on the patient's clinical status (i.e., more for excessive GI loss, nephrotoxic medications, etc. and less for compromised organ function and iatrogenic fluid overload)
   b. Maintenance fluid needs for adults is 1,500 mL/m^2 body surface area

    Oral nutrition should be encouraged as much as possible throughout the transplant process. Autologous transplant patients and some allogeneic transplant patients may be able to maintain adequate oral intake and avoid parenteral nutrition during the transplant period with attention to symptom management. Symptom control via medication or adjustment to diet may help the patient avoid TPN and maintain adequate oral intake. However, the majority of allogeneic transplant patients and those with severe mucositis will require TPN to maintain positive nitrogen balance and prevent significant weight loss.

7.3 USE OF TOTAL PARENTERAL NUTRITION

Patients who are undergoing HSCT with myeloablative conditioning regimens have a higher incidence of various oral and GI complications. Examples of these complications can include, but are not limited to, oral/esophageal mucositis, anorexia, and nausea/vomiting/diarrhea (see Chapter 18). These complications can impair nutritional status by limiting oral intake in the immediate post-transplant period. It is common practice to utilize parenteral nutrition during this period for these patients.

1. TPN Initiation Guidelines
   a. TPN should be considered if the following conditions exist:
      i. Weight loss of ≤5% of usual body weight
      ii. Patient unable to consume at least 50% of basal energy expenditure (BEE) for ≥3 days
      iii. Negligible oral intake (or <50% of BEE) is anticipated for at least seven consecutive days
      iv. Severe gastrointestinal toxicity lasting >5 days is expected with the preparative regimen (e.g., busulfan, etoposide, melphalan, and/or total body irradiation combinations)
   b. Recommend a baseline of 25–30 kcal/kg/day, 1.5 g protein/kg/day, and 20–30% of kcal from lipids
      i. Adjusted body weight should be used for patients ≥125% ideal weight
      ii. Calories and protein provided should be adjusted based on patient's medical condition (i.e., renal failure, fluid status, etc.)
      iii. Lipids are not contraindicated in HSCT patients unless the patient has excessive hypertriglyceridemia, turbid serum or poor clearance
   c. Additional vitamin C (500 mg/day) should be provided to promote tissue recovery via collagen biosynthesis
   d. Additional zinc should be added to TPN for patients with diarrhea at a dose of 1 mg/100 mL
   e. For patients with persistent hyperbilirubinemia (serum bilirubin >10 mg/dL), the trace elements of copper and manganese should be removed from TPN
2. TPN Administration Recommendations
   a. When oral caloric intake is >50% of caloric needs × two consecutive days, discontinue TPN
   b. Taper TPN to 50% of caloric needs as soon as possible to stimulate appetite when oral intake resumes (minimum kcal in TPN will be 1,000/day)
   c. Discontinue TPN at least 1 day prior to anticipated discharge to ensure adequate oral intake
   d. If prolonged nutritional support is anticipated, enteral feeds should be considered in patients who have resolution of severe mucositis, esophagitis, and/or diarrhea

7.4 EXPLANATION OF CATABOLIC/ANABOLIC STATES

An anabolic state is part of the metabolic process where an individual builds muscle mass and loses fat mass, achieved with adequate nutrition and exercise. Multiple factors may prevent achieving anabolic status by cancer patients, including a general systemic effect, a local effect (depending on tumor location), and the type of therapy used to treat the cancer. Despite a patient consuming what appears to be an adequate amount of nutrients, they still may not be able to maintain a state of anabolism due to alterations in host metabolism, inefficiency of nutrient use or the malignancy, and the host competing for nutrients.

The catabolic process occurs when the body needs to break down its own tissue for energy use because there is not enough energy available in the form of food. During times of illness and stress, as in those with an active disease process such as cancer, the body's response is both hypermetabolic and hypercatabolic. The tissue catabolism that happens during this time is mediated through cytokine and counterregulatory hormone release. If left uncorrected, the process of catabolism can lead to loss of lean body mass, which can impair the ability to recover from illness due to the need for protein synthesis for recovery.

Tissue catabolism in cancer patients is likely a factor of inadequate energy intake, hypermetabolism, or both. While hypermetabolism is not present in all patients with cancer, a significant correlation between the disease duration and hypermetabolism has been shown. Recently, data has suggested that hypermetabolism in cancer patients can be related to tumor-induced changes in host hormones, neuropeptides, cytokines, and neurotransmitters, which can have negative effects on appetite and increase protein breakdown (catabolism).

7.5 DISCUSSION OF GLUTAMINE CONTROVERSY

Glutamine, normally a non-essential amino acid, is important in many metabolic processes including proliferation of lymphocytes, macrophages, and fuel for enterocytes, as well as preserving the integrity of the GI mucosa and function of the intestines. The body may not be able to synthesize adequate amounts of glutamine in times of severe physiological stress causing a deficiency and thus may require supplementation of glutamine either oral or IV.

In regards to IV glutamine, the ASPEN Clinical Guidelines have concluded, "pharmacologic doses of parenteral glutamine may benefit patients undergoing hematopoietic cell transplantation". It should be noted that parenteral glutamine is not readily available by US FDA manufacturer process, but instead as a prescription prepared by a compounding pharmacy. In three separate meta-analyses of using IV glutamine, the conclusion was the same; IV glutamine could possibly decrease the number of blood stream infections. There was no benefit with regards to length of stay, time on TPN, or improvement in morbidity/mortality. Oral glutamine has been shown to decrease the incidence or severity of mucositis in patients undergoing HSCT. Despite these positive reports, these particular studies have been small and drug dosing and administration were inconsistent. More studies of glutamine supplementation, either IV or oral, are needed to determine the benefit in the transplant population.

References

August, D., Huhmann, M. (2009). A.S.P.E.N. clinical guidelines: Nutrition support therapy during adult anticancer treatment and in hematopoietic cell transplantation. *J Parent Enter Nutr*, 33(5): 472–500.

Charuhas, P.M. (2006). Medical nutrition therapy in hematopoietic cell transplantation. In L. Elliott, L. Molseed, P. McCallum (Eds.), *The Clinical Guide to Onocology Nutrition* (pp. 126–137). American Dietetic Association, Chicago.

Crowther, M., Avenell, A., Culligan, D.J. (2009). Systematic review and meta-analyses of studies of glutamine supplementation in haematopoietic stem cell transplantation. *Bone Marrow Transplant*, 44(7):413–425.

DeMille, D., Deming, P., Lupinacci, P., Jacobs, L. (2006). The effect of the neutropenic diet in the outpatient setting: A pilot study. *Oncol Nurs Forum*, 33(2):337–343.

Diana, F., Crowther, M. (2009). Symposium 4: Hot topics in parenteral nutrition. A Review of the use of gluatmine supplementation in the nutrition support of patients undergoing bone-marrow transplantation and traditional cancer therapy. *Proc Nutr Soc*, 68(3):269–273.

Dickson, T.M., Wong, R.M., Negrin, R.S., Shizuru, J.A., Johnston, L.J., Hu, W.W., et al. (2000). Effect of oral glutamine supplementation during bone marrow transplantation. *J Parent Enter Nutr*, 24(2): 61–66.

French, M. Levy-Milne R. (2001). A survey of the use of low microbial diets in pediatric bone marrow transplant programs. *J Amer Diet Assoc*, 101(10):1194–1198.

Kuhn, K.S., Muscaritoli, M., Wischmeyer, P., Stehle, P. (2010). Glutamine as indispensable nutrient in oncology: Experimental and clinical evidence. *Eur J Nutr*, 49(4):197–210.

Moody, K., Charlson, M., Finlay, J. (2002). The neutropenic diet: What's the evidence. *J Pediatric Hematol Oncol*, 24(9):717–721.

Murray, S., S, P. (2009). Nutrition support for bone marrow tranplant patients. *Cochrane Database of Syst Rev*, 1.

Nirenberg, A., Bush, A.P., Dvais, A., Friese, C., Gillespie, T., Rice, R.D. (2006). Neutropenia: State of the knowledge part II. *Oncol Nursing Forum*, 33(6):1202–1208.

Nutritional assessment methods. (2002). In P.M. Charuhas (Ed.), *Hematopoietic Stem Cell Transplantation Nutrition Care Criteria* (2nd ed., p. 44). The Fred Hutchinson Cancer Research Center, Seattle, Washington.

Recommendations of CDC. (2000, October 20). *Guidelines for preventing opportunistic infections Among Hematopoietic Stem Cell Transplant Recipients*. (CDC, Editor) Retrieved February 17, 2010, from http://www.cdc.gov/mmwr/preview/mmwrhtml/rr4910al.htm: http://www.cdc.gov/mmwr/preview/mmwrhtml/rr4910al.htm

Restau, J., Clark, A. (2008). The neutropenic diet: Does the evidence support this intervention. *Clin Nurse Spec*, 22(5):208–211.

Roberts, S., Mattox, T. (2007). Cancer. In M.M. Gottschlich (Ed.), *The A.S.P.E.N. Nutrition Support Core Curriculum* (2nd ed., pp. 652–653). ASPEN, Silver Spring, MD.

Skop, A., Kolarzyk, E., Skotnicki, A. (2005). Importance of parenteral nutrition in patients undergoing hematopoietic stem cell transplantation procedures in the autologous system. *J Parent Enter Nutr*, 29(4):241–247.

Wolfe, B.M. (1991). Nutrition in hypermetabolic conditions. In F. Zeman (Ed.), *Clincial Nutrition and Dietetics* (2nd ed., p. 557). Macmillan Publishing Company, Englewood Cliffs.

Wooley, J.A., Frankenfield, D. (2007). Energy. In M.M. Gottschlich (Ed.), *The A.S.P.E.N. Nutrition Support Core Curriculum* (2nd ed., pp. 20–21) ASPEN, Silver Spring, MD.

Zeman, F. (1991). Nutrition and cancer. In F. Zeman (Ed.), *Clincial Nutrition and Dietetics* (2nd ed., pp. 577–578). Macmillan Publishing Company, Englewood Cliffs.

CHAPTER 8
Infection Prophylaxis

Lynne Strasfeld

Infections remain an important cause of non-relapse mortality in HSCT recipients. Specific risk for infection is related to prior exposure history (e.g., relapse of latent infection), intensity of conditioning regimens and immunosuppression, and new exposures in the setting of altered host immune response. Prevention of infection by prophylactic and preemptive strategies has been associated with improvement in transplant outcomes over the past few decades. The introduction of new oral antivirals (e.g., valganciclovir) and antifungal compounds (e.g., posaconazole, voriconazole) in the past decade has allowed for a less toxic and more facile approach to infection prevention.

8.1 HERPES SIMPLEX VIRUS (HSV)/VARICELLA ZOSTER VIRUS (VZV) PROPHYLAXIS

1. HSV and VZV reactivation is common in the absence of antiviral prophylaxis. The duration and dose of acyclovir [or valacyclovir] prophylaxis varies by host serostatus and transplant type. See Table 8.1.
2. If nausea or mucositis precludes oral intake, change to IV acyclovir until patient is able to tolerate oral intake. If oral acyclovir is unavailable, valacyclovir is an option for prophylaxis. For dosing recommendations, see Table 8.2.
3. If patient develops overt signs of oral or genital mucocutaneous HSV infection while on prophylactic dosing, increase dose to 5 mg/kg IV q8 h of acyclovir or treatment doses

R.T. Maziarz, S. Slater (eds.), *Blood and Marrow Transplant Handbook*, DOI 10.1007/978-1-4419-7506-5_8, © Springer Science+Business Media, LLC 2011

TABLE 8.1. HSV/VZV prophylaxis indication and duration

	VZV–/HSV–	VZV–/HSV+	VZV+/HSV–/+
Autologous	No prophylaxis required	Acyclovir (or valacyclovir) through day +100	Acyclovir (or valacyclovir) through day +365
Allogeneic	No prophylaxis required	Acyclovir (or valacyclovir) until off all immune suppression	Acyclovir (or valacyclovir) through day +365 or off all immune suppression

TABLE 8.2. Dosing recommendations for acyclovir, valacyclovir

		Normal renal function	Renal impairment	
		CrCl $\geq$50 mL/min	CrCl 30–49 mL/min	CrCl <30 mL/min
Acyclovir PO	Autologous	800 mg po daily	800 mg po daily	400 mg po daily
	Allogeneic	800 mg po BID	800 mg po daily	400 mg po daily
Valacyclovir PO	Autologous	500 mg po daily	500 mg po daily	500 mg po daily
	Allogeneic	500 mg po BID	500 mg po daily	500 mg po daily
Acyclovir IV	Autologous or allogeneic	250 mg/m^2 IV q12h	250 mg/m^2 IV q24h	250 mg IV q24h

of oral acyclovir (400 mg po 5×/day) or valacyclovir (500–1,000 mg po BID). If symptoms persist despite therapeutic doses of acyclovir, send HSV culture and consider the possibility of acyclovir-resistant HSV, which would entail treatment with foscarnet.

4. VZV-seronegative immunocompromised allogeneic HSCT recipients (<24 months post-transplant, >24 months post-transplant and on immunosuppressive therapy, or with chronic GVHD) with close contact with a person with either primary varicella (chickenpox) or herpes zoster (shingles) should receive varicella zoster-specific immunoglobulin as

soon as possible and within 96 h of the exposure. VariZIG is currently available only by way of an expanded access protocol (Cangene Corporation, Winnipeg, Canada).

5. Family members and close contacts who receive the Varivax or Zostavax vaccine and develop a rash after vaccination should avoid contact with the transplant recipient.

6. If a hospitalized transplant patient develops varicella zoster infection (either primary infection or reactivation infection with or without dissemination), they should be placed in contact and airborne precautions and moved to a negative airflow room. Consider placement off the transplant ward.

8.2 CYTOMEGALOVIRUS (CMV) MONITORING AND PREEMPTIVE THERAPY

1. Autologous patients*: No CMV surveillance is required unless clinically indicated (e.g., patients with protracted fevers, GI symptoms). If patient has documented CMV disease within 1 year prior to autologous transplant of CD34$^+$ selected PBSC product, weekly CMV PCRs should be followed through day +100.

   a. *CMV-seropositive autologous recipients who have received major T-cell suppression within 6 months of transplant (e.g., alemtuzumab, fludarabine, or 2-chlorodeoxyadenosine), patients receiving total body irradiation as part of the conditioning regimen, and patients who receive T-cell-depleted grafts are at risk for symptomatic CMV infection or disease and should have preemptive monitoring through at least day +60.

2. Allogeneic patients

   a. All allogeneic patients who are CMV-seropositive or have a CMV-seropositive donor should have weekly serum CMV quantitative PCRs beginning on transplant admission and through day +100, then thereafter every other week if steroid dose is >10 mg/day.

   b. Patients who are CMV-seronegative with a CMV-seronegative donor should have monthly CMV PCR, surveillance through day +100.

3. Any patient with CMV infection prior to or after day +100 should have prolonged surveillance

   a. If no GvHD is present, continue surveillance weekly for 3 months following infection, then every other week for 3 months.

    b. If GvHD is present, continue surveillance weekly for 1 year following infection

4. Triggers to begin preemptive therapy include two consecutive "weak positive" (detectable but less than 200 copies/mL, the cutoff for quantification) CMV quantitative PCRs or a single quantitative PCR with a quantifiable copy number. Prophylactic acyclovir should be stopped if preemptive therapy for CMV infection is initiated.

5. Oral valganciclovir can be used as preemptive therapy for any patient without signs/symptoms suggestive of CMV end-organ disease and meeting the all of the following criteria:

    a. No signs/symptoms or suspicion of CMV end-organ disease

        i. Negative chest X-ray (chest X-ray should be performed at time of documentation of CMV infection, with finer imaging reserved for symptomatic presentation)

        ii. Absence of gastrointestinal complaints (nausea, vomiting, diarrhea)

        iii. Afebrile

        iv. No evidence of other end-organ manifestations of CMV infection: hepatitis, retinitis, encephalitis, myelosuppression

    b. Viral load <5,000 copies/mL

    c. No history of medication noncompliance

    d. Able to tolerate adequate oral intake/medications

    e. No evidence of gut GvHD

6. Preemptive valganciclovir dosing is 900 mg po BID until quantitative PCRs are negative × 2 weeks, then 900 mg po daily × 14 days (induction/maintenance dosing, renal dose adjustment as outlined in Table 8.3). Valganciclovir should be taken with food. If quantitative PCR remains negative, discontinue valganciclovir and resume prophylactic acyclovir.

7. If CMV viral load continues to rise after 14 days of therapy, change to high-dose IV ganciclovir and consider the unlikely possibility of ganciclovir-resistant CMV. In this setting, consultation with the Infectious Diseases Service is advised. If concern for ganciclovir-resistance is sufficiently high, resistance testing (typically by genotypic analysis) can be done, with consideration for an empiric switch to foscarnet in patients who develop life-or sight-threatening disease (see point 4 in Section 14.4).

TABLE 8.3. Valganciclovir dosing in renal impairment

CrCl	Normal renal function	Renal impairment[a]			
	≥60 mL/min	40–59 mL/min	25–39 mL/min	10–24 mL/min	<10 mL/min (hemodialysis)
Induction	900 mg po BID	450 mg po BID	450 mg po daily	450 mg po QOD	DO NOT USE
Maintenance	900 mg po daily	450 mg po daily	450 mg po QOD	450 mg po twice weekly	DO NOT USE

[a]Patients with renal insufficiency whose CMV reactivates should receive valganciclovir 900 mg po BID × 2 doses. The dose should then be adjusted for their renal function as outlined above

8. If the patient does not meet the criteria outlined above in point 5 in Section 8.2, CMV preemptive therapy should consist of ganciclovir 5 mg/kg IV BID until quantitative PCRs are negative × 2 weeks, then 5 mg/kg IV daily × 14 days (induction/maintenance dosing, renal dose adjustment as outlined in Table 8.4). If PCRs remain negative, discontinue ganciclovir and resume prophylactic acyclovir.

9. If CMV reactivation occurs after day +100, decision to treat preemptively will depend on height of circulating viral load as well as host immune status. Preemptive treatment should be with either oral valganciclovir or IV ganciclovir as directed above. Continue therapy until patient with negative PCR on two consecutive weeks.

10. Given the poor outcomes associated with CMV disease prior to allogeneic transplantation, patients with documented pre-transplant CMV infections warrant special consideration with regard to preemptive monitoring strategies, and even consideration for prophylaxis in some settings.

8.3 ANTIBACTERIAL PROPHYLAXIS

1. Autologous and allogeneic recipients should receive fluoro-quirolane prophylaxis (e.g., levofloxacin 500 mg po daily or ciprofloxacin 500 mg po BID) from day −1 until ANC >500/mm^3 on two consecutive days or until first neutropenic temperature spike (temperature ≥38°C) occurs, at which time empiric broad spectrum parenteral antibiotic therapy is begun (see Chapter 14) after appropriate cultures obtained.

2. If patient is unable to tolerate oral medications, use IV formulation of quinolone (levofloxacin 500 mg IV daily or ciprofloxacin 400 mg IV BID).

3. In the case of a documented quinolone allergy, IV ceftazidime or cefepime can be considered an alternative.

8.4 ENCAPSULATED ORGANISM PROPHYLAXIS FOR PATIENTS WITH CHRONIC GVHD

1. All patients with chronic GvHD and all asplenic patients should receive prophylaxis for encapsulated organisms with oral penicillin VK 500 mg po daily.

2. Alternatives for patients who are penicillin-allergic include

TABLE 8.4. Ganciclovir dosing in renal impairment[a]

	Normal renal function	Renal impairment			
CrCl	$\geq$70 mL/min	50–69 mL/min	25–49 mL/min	10–24 mL/min	<10 mL/min (hemodialysis)
Induction	5 mg/kg IV q12 h	2.5–5 mg/kg IV q 12 h	2.5 mg/kg IV q 24 h	1.25 mg/kg IV q 24 h	1.25–2.5 mg/kg IV 3×/week (dose following dialysis)
Maintenance	5 mg/kg IV q 24 h	2.5 mg/kg IV q 24 h	1.25 mg/kg IV q 24 h	0.625 mg/kg IV q 24 h	0.625 mg/kg IV 3×/week (dose following dialysis)

[a]Patients with renal insufficiency whose CMV reactivates should receive ganciclovir 5 mg/kg IV q 12 h × 2 doses. The dose should then be adjusted for their renal function as outlined above

a. Azithromycin 250 mg po daily (in particular in patients with chronic bronchiolitis obliterans)
b. Trimethoprim/sulfamethoxazole single strength 1 tablet po daily

8.5 ANTIFUNGAL PROPHYLAXIS

1. Autologous patients should receive fluconazole 400 mg po/IV daily beginning day 0 and continuing through day +30 at least, with consideration of continuation until day +75.
2. Allogeneic patients should receive fluconazole 400 mg po/IV daily beginning day 0 and continuing until day +75 for nonmyeloablative transplants or day +100 for myeloablative transplants.
   a. Weekly galactomannan assays should be monitored, and patients will be evaluated for invasive aspergillosis (inclusive of a CT scan of the chest) if the assay is positive, with strong consideration for change to voriconazole while work-up is underway.
   b. Alternatives to fluconazole prophylaxis (if dose-limiting liver function test abnormalities, documented allergy, or significant drug–drug interactions) include an echinocandin, e.g., micafungin 100 mg IV daily or liposomal amphotericin B products 1 mg/kg IV daily or 3 mg/kg three times weekly.
3. Patients who receive high-dose steroids after transplant ($\geq$0.4 mg/kg/day of methylprednisolone equivalent) for treatment of acute or chronic GvHD or for other indications (e.g., idiopathic pneumonia syndrome, diffuse alveolar hemorrhage, etc.) should receive posaconazole prophylaxis (see Table 8.5 for azole dosing).
   a. If enteral absorption problematic or if oral intake insufficient, change posaconazole prophylaxis to voriconazole.
   b. Alternatives to extended-spectrum azole prophylaxis (if dose-limiting liver function test abnormalities, documented allergy, QT_c prolongation, or significant drug–drug interactions) include liposomal amphotericin B products 1 mg/kg IV daily or 3 mg/kg three times weekly (with close monitoring of renal function) or an echinocandin, e.g., micafungin 100 mg IV daily, though noting echinocandin therapy is less optimal given the risk for breakthrough mold infection.

TABLE 8.5. Azole dosing

Drug	Adult dose	
Fluconazole	400 mg po/IV daily[a]	
Posaconazole[b,c]	200 mg po TID	Dose with meals and ensure no proton-pump inhibitor/H2-blocker therapy to maximize absorption
Voriconazole[b,d]	6 mg/kg IV q 12 × 2 doses (loading dose), then 4 mg/kg po/IV q 12 (maintenance)	Oral dosing on an empty stomach to maximize absorption

[a] Renal dose adjustment required, dose at 200 mg daily for CrCl <50 mL/min

[b] Extended spectrum azoles are metabolized primarily by cytochrome P450 enzymes, and as such there are numerous critical drug–drug interactions to be mindful of, including by not limited to the calcineurin inhibitors and sirolimus as well as multiple chemotherapeutic agents. Consult package insert, Bruggemann et al. (*Clin Infect Dis* 2009;48:1441–1458.), transplant pharmacist, and/or Infectious Diseases consultation service before prescribing these medications

[c] Posaconazole levels can vary and monitoring of levels should be considered if breakthrough fungal infection occurs or if suspected toxicity (liver function test abnormalities)

[d] Voriconazole levels can vary and monitoring of levels should be considered in patients with suspected toxicity (liver function test abnormalities and/or confusion/delirium), if breakthrough fungal infection, or if therapeutic failure

8.6 PNEUMOCYSTIS JIROVECI (PCP) PROPHYLAXIS

1. All patients should receive trimethoprim/sulfamethoxazole DS 1 tablet po BID beginning the first day of their conditioning regimen, continuing through day –2.

2. Both autologous and allogeneic patients should resume PCP prophylaxis between days +30 and +40. Standard prophylaxis is trimethoprim/sulfamethoxazole DS 1 tablet po BID twice weekly. Alternatives in the sulfa-allergic patient include*

   a. Dapsone 100 mg po daily (consider checking G-6PD level prior to initiation of dapsone)

b. Pentamidine 4 mg/kg IV or 300 mg aerosolized q4 weeks

c. Atovaquone 1,500 mg po daily

3. PCP prophylaxis should continue for a total of 6 months for autologous recipients and until discontinuation of all immunosuppressive therapy in allogeneic recipients.

* Keep in mind there is no Toxoplasma prophylaxis with agents other than trimethoprim/sulfamethoxazole.

8.7 VANCOMYCIN-RESISTANT ENTEROCOCCUS (VRE) SURVEILLANCE AND CONTACT ISOLATION PROCEDURES

VRE colonization/infection is a growing problem in hospitalized patients, and is associated with poor outcomes in HSCT recipients, with a significant percentage of patients with colonization progressing to systemic infection. In the context of VRE transmission on a HSCT unit, an active surveillance program can be considered. An example of our hospital's institutional policy is provided below.

1. All patients with a history of VRE colonization or infection are maintained on contact isolation for the duration of the hospital stay and for visits to the outpatient transplant clinic.

2. Patients not previously known to be VRE-colonized or infected are placed in contact isolation at the time of hospital admission and a rectal swab for VRE PCR obtained.

   a. If the rectal VRE PCR is negative, contact isolation can be discontinued and weekly surveillance continued during the course of hospitalization.

   b. If the rectal VRE PCR is positive, the patient will be placed on contact isolation until de-escalation of isolation is appropriate (see below).

3. In a patient with a history of VRE colonization or infection, attempt at de-escalation of isolation precautions can be pursued when:

   a. Last detection of VRE by PCR or culture is >3 months prior

   b. Patient has been off of systemic antibiotic therapy for at least 3 weeks and is clinically stable

4. VRE isolation precautions can be discontinued in a patient with documented history of VRE colonization or infection when the conditions outlined above (point 3 in Section 7) are satisfied and when three consecutive rectal swabs (separated in time by at least 7 days) for VRE PCR are negative.

References

A new product (VariZIG) for postexposure prophylaxis of varicella available under an investigational new drug application expanded access protocol. (2006). *MMWR Morb Mortal Wkly Rep,* 55:209–210.

Ayala, E., Greene, J., Sandin, R., et al. (2006). Valganciclovir is safe and effective as pre-emptive therapy for CMV infection in allogeneic hematopoietic stem cell transplantation. *Bone Marrow Transplant,* 37:851–856.

Boeckh, M., Ljungman, P. (2009). How we treat cytomegalovirus in hematopoietic cell transplant recipients. *Blood,* 113:5711–5719.

Busca, A., de Fabritiis, P., Ghisetti, V., et al. (2007). Oral valganciclovir as preemptive therapy for cytomegalovirus infection post allogeneic stem cell transplantation. *Transpl Infect Dis,* 9:102–107.

Bruggemann, R.J., Alffenaar, J.W., Blijlevens, N.M., et al. (2009). Clinical relevance of the pharmacokinetic interactions of azole antifungal drugs with other coadministered agents. *Clin Infect Dis,* 48:1441–1458.

Einsele, H., Reusser, P., Bornhauser, M., et al. (2006). Oral valganciclovir leads to higher exposure to ganciclovir than intravenous ganciclovir in patients following allogeneic stem cell transplantation. *Blood,* 107:3002–3008.

Fries, B.C., Riddell, S.R., Kim, H.W., et al. (2005). Cytomegalovirus disease before hematopoietic cell transplantation as a risk for complications after transplantation. *Biol Blood Marrow Transplant,* 11:136–148.

Holmberg, L.A., Boeckh, M., Hooper, H., et al. (1999). Increased incidence of cytomegalovirus disease after autologous CD34-selected peripheral blood stem cell transplantation. *Blood,* 94:4029–4035.

Madureira, A., Bergeron, A., Lacroix, C., et al. (2007). Breakthrough invasive aspergillosis in allogeneic haematopoietic stem cell transplant recipients treated with caspofungin. *Int J Antimicrob Agents,* 30:551–554.

Marr, K.A., Seidel, K., Slavin, M.A., et al. (2000). Prolonged fluconazole prophylaxis is associated with persistent protection against candidiasis-related death in allogeneic marrow transplant recipients: long-term follow-up of a randomized, placebo-controlled trial. *Blood,* 96:2055–2061.

Muto, C.A., Jernigan, J.A., Ostrowsky, B.E., et al. (2003). SHEA guideline for preventing nosocomial transmission of multidrug-resistant strains of staphylococcus aureus and enterococcus. *Infect Control Hosp Epidemiol,* 24:362–386.

Tomblyn, M., Chiller, T., Einsele, H., et al. (2009). Guidelines for preventing infectious complications among hematopoietic cell transplantation recipients: a global perspective. *Biol Blood Marrow Transplant,* 15:1143–1238.

Ullmann, A.J., Lipton, J.H., Vesole, D.H., et al. (2007) Posaconazole or fluconazole for prophylaxis in severe graft-versus-host disease. *N Engl J Med,* 356:335–347.

van Burik, J.A., Ratanatharathorn, V., Stepan, D.E., et al. (2004). Micafungin versus fluconazole for prophylaxis against invasive fungal infections during neutropenia in patients undergoing hematopoietic stem cell transplantation. *Clin Infect Dis*, 39:1407–1416.

van der Heiden, P.L., Kalpoe, J.S., Barge, R.M., Willemze, R., Kroes, A.C., Schippers, E.F. (2006). Oral valganciclovir as pre-emptive therapy has similar efficacy on cytomegalovirus DNA load reduction as intravenous ganciclovir in allogeneic stem cell transplantation recipients. *Bone Marrow Transplant*, 37:693–698.

Weinstock, D.M., Conlon, M., Iovino, C., et al. (2007). Colonization, bloodstream infection, and mortality caused by vancomycin-resistant enterococcus early after allogeneic hematopoietic stem cell transplant. *Biol Blood Marrow Transplant*, 13:615–621.

Zirakzadeh, A., Gastineau, D.A., Mandrekar, J.N., Burke, J.P., Johnston, P.B., Patel, R. (2008). Vancomycin-resistant enterococcal colonization appears associated with increased mortality among allogeneic hematopoietic stem cell transplant recipients. *Bone Marrow Transplant*, 41:385–392.

CHAPTER 9
Graft-Versus-Host Disease Prophylaxis

Erin Corella

The development of acute graft-versus-host disease (GvHD) has been proposed to be the consequence of a chain of events. First, the host environment is damaged by the transplant conditioning regimen. As a result, pro-inflammatory cytokines such as tumor necrosis factor and interleukins are released and host antigen-presenting cells (APCs) are activated. Second, donor T cells are recruited along with other inflammatory cells to the area and are activated when they bind to host APCs by recognizing alterations of "self" expressed on the major histocompatibility complex (MHC) molecules. Once donor T-cells proliferate and differentiate, they contribute to further tissue damage to the host, most commonly seen in the skin, gut, and liver. While there is ongoing research looking at the utility of donor T-cell depletion, this section will focus on the immunosuppressive agents used post-transplantation to suppress host inflammatory response and donor T-cell activation.

9.1 STANDARD REGIMENS
1. Myeloablative transplant
   a. Cyclosporine/methotrexate
   b. Tacrolimus/methotrexate
   c. Cyclosporine/methotrexate/methylprednisolone
   d. Other prophylaxis regimens may be dictated by clinical trials
      i. Tacrolimus/sirolimus
2. Nonmyeloablative transplant
   a. Cyclosporine/methotrexate
   b. Tacrolimus/methotrexate

R.T. Maziarz, S. Slater (eds.), *Blood and Marrow Transplant Handbook*, DOI 10.1007/978-1-4419-7506-5_9, © Springer Science+Business Media, LLC 2011

c. Cyclosporine/mycophenolate mofetil
d. Other prophylaxis regimens may be dictated by clinical trials
  i. Tacrolimus/mycophenolate mofetil
  ii. Tacrolimus/sirolimus

9.2 AGENTS USED FOR GVHD PROPHYLAXIS

1. Cyclosporine and tacrolimus
   a. Mechanism of action/place in therapy
      i. Inhibit calcineurin resulting in a decreased production of IL-2. IL-2 is one of the major cytokines responsible for activation and proliferation of T cells.
      ii. Commonly used in conjunction with methotrexate for prevention of GVHD in myeloablative transplants and in conjunction with mycophenolate for prevention of GVHD in nonmyeloablative transplants.
   b. Dose and administration
      i. Cyclosporine in myeloablative transplants
         – Continuous infusion
            1. 3 mg/kg/day IV beginning day −1
            2. May begin with 5 mg/kg/day IV from day −1 to day +3 before converting to 3 mg/kg/day
         – Bolus dosing:
            1. IV: 1.5–2 mg/kg/dose IV every 12 h beginning day −2. Infuse over 2–4 h.
      ii. Cyclosporine in nonmyeloablative transplants
         – Continuous infusion
            1. 3 mg/kg/day IV beginning anywhere from day −3 to day −1
            2. May begin with 1 mg/kg/day IV from day −7 to day −2 before converting to 3 mg/kg/day on day −1
         – Bolus dosing:
            1. PO: 4 mg/kg/dose PO every 12 h beginning day −3
      iii. Tacrolimus in myeloablative transplants
         – Continuous infusion
            1. 0.02–0.03 mg/kg/day IV beginning anywhere from day −3 to day −1
         – Bolus dosing
            1. IV: 0.015 mg/kg/dose IV every 12 h beginning day −1. Infuse over 2–4 h.

    2. PO: 0.05–0.075 mg/kg/dose PO every 12 h beginning day −1

iv. Tacrolimus in nonmyeloablative transplants
- Bolus dosing

    1. PO: 0.025–0.03 mg/kg/dose PO every 12 h beginning day −3

v. Conversion from IV to PO
- Cyclosporine: Convert to PO agent using an IV:PO conversion factor of 1:1.8 or 1:2. Gengraf® or equivalent is preferable.
- Tacrolimus: Convert to PO as soon as possible using an IV:PO conversion factor of 1:3 or 1:4

vi. Conversion from cyclosporine to tacrolimus
- Monitor daily cyclosporine levels and begin tacrolimus when cyclosporine level is <100–125 ng/mL to decrease the renal toxicity associated with this drug combination.
- Begin tacrolimus at 1/3 the normal starting dose and titrate up slowly if using in conjunction with an azole antifungal.

vii. Tapering doses
- Tapering schedule varies based on protocol and institutional standards. Day of taper initiation and duration of therapy varies from center to center.
- General rules

    1. Taper dose approximately 5–10% each week if no active GVHD is observed

    2. Begin taper at approximately day +100 with a plan to discontinue drug by day +365 for ablative transplant recipients

    3. Taper for nonmyeloablative transplant recipients begins at day +56, tapered by 6% weekly with a goal of tapering off by day +180

viii. Other information
- Hold cyclosporine or tacrolimus dose on day 0 if scheduled within 4 h of stem cell infusion.
- Cyclosporine IV is usually given as bolus doses. Patients may experience an increased rate of acute GVHD grade II–IV when cyclosporine is given as a continuous IV infusion. However, continuous infusion may confer better disease-free survival in high-risk patients.

- There is no statistically significant benefit to administering cyclosporine for 24 months versus 6 months with regard to development of chronic GVHD.
- Tacrolimus IV is usually given as a continuous infusion rather than bolus doses due to increased renal and neurologic toxicity seen with bolus doses.

c. Monitoring
  i. Trough concentrations vary based on protocol and institutional standards.
  ii. Trough concentrations
    - Cyclosporine in myeloablative transplants: 150–450 ng/mL. Usual range is 200–300 ng/mL.
    - Cyclosporine in nonmyeloablative transplants: 100–400 ng/mL. Higher concentrations early post-transplant may be warranted with some conditioning regimens to maximize immune suppression
      1. Day –3 through day +28: 300–400 ng/mL
      2. Day +29 through day +56: 250–350 ng/mL
    - Tacrolimus in myeloablative transplants: 5–20 ng/mL. Usual range is 5–10 ng/mL.
    - Tacrolimus in nonmyeloablative transplants: 5–20 ng/mL. Usual range is 5–15 ng/mL.
  iii. Checking levels:
    - Levels are to be checked no sooner than 36 h following a change in dose or schedule (at least three doses if given every 12 h).
    - Routine monitoring of levels should occur twice a week, early in HSCT course.
    - If giving drug by continuous infusion, hold infusion for a minimum of 15 min prior to collecting level and draw level from lumen of catheter that is not used for infusion of calcineurin inhibitor.
  iv. Other information
    - IV infusions should always occur through the same IV line. An alternate site should be used for collecting trough levels.
    - Patient will have a spuriously high level if sample is drawn from line used for infusion. Draw an additional level from a peripheral stick to confirm the accuracy of an abnormally high level.
    - Achieving target cyclosporine concentrations in the second week of transplant and the week prior

TABLE 9.1. Dose adjustment for renal insufficiency

Creatinine (mg/dL)	Cyclosporine/tacrolimus taper
1.5–1.75 (or 1–1.5× baseline)	50–75% of current dose
1.76–2 (or 1.6–1.9× baseline)	25–50% of current dose
>2.0 (or >1.9 × baseline)	Hold until creatinine <2.0, then resume at 50–75% of prior dose

to engraftment will significantly reduce the chance of developing acute GVHD.

d. Dose adjustments

   i. Adjust doses by 10–15% each time serum levels are outside of goal range.

   ii. Adjust doses by up to 30% each time depending on severity of hepatic insufficiency.

   iii. Adjust doses for renal insufficiency (see Table 9.1).

     – The risk of creatinine >2× baseline increases by 94% when the mean concentration of cyclosporine is >300 for 7–14 days.

     – The risk of creatinine >2× baseline increases by 41% when the mean concentration of tacrolimus is >20 for 7–14 days.

     – Withholding a single dose of the calcineurin inhibitor prior to re-institution of the lower dose can assist in the dose modification effort.

   iv. Dose adjust for drug interactions with CYP 3A4 Inhibitors such as amiodarone, azole antifungals, calcium channel blockers, nicardipine, macrolide antibiotics, protease inhibitors, and some tyrosine kinase inhibitors.

     – Depending on the strength of azole antifungal as an inhibitor, cyclosporine doses may need to be reduced as much as 60% when given concomitantly with the azole.

     – Adjust doses by up to 20% each time.

   v. Adjust dose for drug interactions with CYP 3A4 inducers such as carbamazepine, phenobarbital, phenytoin, rifabutin, rifampin.

e. Adverse effects (note: There is no strict correlation between toxicity and level)

i. Adverse effects common to cyclosporine and tacrolimus:
   – Hypertension
     • Treat with a calcium channel blocker, such as nifedepine ER (Adalat CC®) or amlodipine (Norvasc®).
     • Avoid ACE inhibitors and ˙ diuretics with cyclosporine. They can exacerbate the already reduced renal blood flow caused by cyclosporine due to afferent arteriole vasoconstriction.
     • It is critically important to maintain DBP <90.
   – Renal impairment
     • Decrease dose to avoid continued damage to kidneys. See dose adjustments in Table 9.1.
   – Electrolyte abnormalities: hypomagnesemia, hyperkalemia
   – Neurotoxicity: tremors, ataxia, headache, seizures
     • Obtain MRI. If posterior leukoencephalopathy is evidenced by MRI, hold doses. The condition is reversible.
     • Treat seizures with antiepileptic agents such as phenytoin or levetiracetam.
     • Reduce tremors with propranolol 10 mg PO every 6 h.
   – Hepatic impairment: hyperbilirubinemia
     • Cyclosporine and tacrolimus are excreted through the bile in feces.
     • Monitor levels closely and decrease dose.
   – Hemolytic uremic syndrome/microangiopathic hemolytic anemia (MAHA)/transplant-associated thrombotic microangiopathy (TATMA) (see Chapter 22)
   – Diabetes
ii. Adverse effects specific to cyclosporine
   – Infusion reaction: burning hands and feet, whole body flushing, and/or muscle cramping
     • May be reaction to the cremaphor diluent.
     • Slow the every 12-h infusion or give the daily dose as a continuous infusion.
     • Premedication with diphenhydramine or oral administration of cyclosporine may be required.
   – Hypertrichosis/hirsutism
   – Gingival hyperplasia
   – Arthralgias and myalgias
     • Can be seen with first dose. Treat with narcotic analgesics.

  iii. Adverse effects specific to tacrolimus
      – Neurotoxicity: hallucinations, nightmares
      – Infusion reaction
          • May be reaction to the castor oil and dehydrated alcohol in the formulation.
          • Premedicate with diphenhydramine and give tacrolimus orally if possible.
2. Methotrexate
  a. Mechanism of action/place in therapy
      i. Inhibits dihydrofolate reductase resulting in a lack of reduced folates available for thymidylate and purine synthesis. As a result, lymphocytes are unable to proliferate.
      ii. Used in conjunction with cyclosporine, tacrolimus, or sirolimus for prevention of GVHD in myeloablative transplants.
  b. Dose and administration
      i. Standard regimen
          – 15 mg/m^2 IV push on day +1. Administer at least 24 h after infusion of stem cells
          – 10 mg/m^2 IV push on day +3, +6 ($\pm$ day +11)
          – Potential benefits of these regimens have been suggested with patients receiving PBSCs demonstrating an increased disease-free and overall survival when given day +11 methotrexate versus those receiving BM and day +11 methotrexate
      ii. Mini-dose
          – 5 mg/m^2 IV push on day +1, +3, +6, +11
      iii. Assess patient prior to each dose and consider holding the dose for third spacing (pleural or pericardial effusions, ascites), liver insufficiency, renal failure, or advanced grade mucositis.
  c. Monitoring
      i. High serum methotrexate levels can be toxic to an early graft
      ii. Check serum methotrexate level 24 h after the dose is given if toxicity is suspected
      iii. May use folinic acid rescue if serum levels are >0.05 micromole/L. Alternatively, when concerned about toxicity, rescue with folinic acid 10 mg IV q 6 h for eight doses, beginning 24 h after the last dose of methotrexate.
  d. Dose adjustments
      i. Dose adjust for liver insufficiency (see Table 9.2)

TABLE 9.2.   Methotrexate dosing in liver insufficiency

Bilirubin (mg/dL)	Methotrexate dose
<3.0	100%
3.1–6.0	50%
>6.0	Hold

  ii. If patient has renal failure/compromise, consider with-holding dose.
 e. Adverse effects
    i. Minimal toxicity at low doses
   ii. Mucositis
      – May hold the dose or decrease to 5 mg/m^2 if grade IV mucositis is present.
      – May use folinic acid rescue 10 mg IV every 6 h for eight doses to prevent exacerbation of existing mucositis. Begin 24 h after administration of methotrexate dose.
      – Use of folinic acid does not affect acute GVHD outcomes.
   iii. Hyperbilirubinemia
    iv. Delayed neutrophil and platelet recovery
3. Corticosteroids
  a. Mechanism of action/place in therapy
    i. Suppresses immune response to stimuli.
   ii. Can be used in conjunction with cyclosporine or tacrolimus and methotrexate for prevention of GVHD in myeloablative transplants.
  b. Dose and administration
    i. Methylprednisolone
      – 0.25 mg/kg/dose IV every 12 h beginning day +7 or day +14
      – Institutional variations in dose schedule may include an increase in dose to 0.5 mg/kg/dose IV every 12 h during weeks 2 and 3 after initiation.
   ii. Conversion from IV to PO
      – Convert to PO prednisone using an IV:PO conversion factor of 1:1.
      – Standard conversion factor is 4:5; however, no loss of efficacy has been observed in practice using 1:1.
   iii. Tapering doses

– Tapering schedule varies based on protocol and institutional standards. Day of taper initiation and duration of therapy varies from center to center.
– General rules
   1. Taper dose approximately 5% each week if no GVHD
   2. Begin taper at approximately day +30 with the goal of reaching 10 mg PO daily by day +84.
   3. Hold prednisone dose at 10 mg PO daily when beginning to taper calcineurin inhibitor at approximately day 100.

c. Monitoring/adverse effects
   i. Diabetes
      – Monitor blood glucose levels on a regular basis and supplement patient with short-acting insulin on an as needed basis and intermediate-acting insulin on a scheduled basis.
   ii. Infection
      – Patients should receive antifungal prophylaxis in the pre-engraftment and post-engraftment transplant periods, and consider long-term use when a patient is taking >30 mg/day of prednisone.

d. Additional Information
   i. The addition of corticosteroids to a prophylaxis regimen will significantly reduce the patient's risk for acute GVHD grade I–II, but does not decrease the incidence of acute GVHD grade III–IV or chronic GVHD.

4. Mycophenolate mofetil
   a. Mechanism of action/place in therapy
      i. Inhibits both T and B lymphocyte proliferation via inhibition of inosine monophosphate dehydrogenase (IMPDH).
      ii. Used in conjunction with cyclosporine and tacrolimus for prevention of GVHD in nonmyeloablative transplants. Replaces methotrexate in 2–3 drug combinations.
   b. Dose and administration
      i. Myeloablative transplants
         – 500–1,500 mg PO/IV 2–3 times daily or 15 mg/kg/dose PO/IV 2–3 times daily beginning day 0 or +1
         – Administration of 15 mg/kg/dose three times daily will provide serum concentrations of

mycophenolate similar to those seen in the solid organ transplant setting.

ii. Nonmyeloablative transplants
   - 1,000 mg PO/IV 2–3 times daily or 15 mg/kg/dose PO/IV 2–3 times daily
   - First dose should be at least 4–6 h after the stem cell infusion.
   - Some institutions will alter mycophenolate dosing based on stem cell source; related donor transplant recipients receive twice daily dosing while unrelated donor transplant recipients receive three times daily dosing.

iii. Conversion from IV to PO
   - Do not crush/open capsules and administer on an empty stomach if possible.
   - Dose can be given as an IV infusion over 2 h if necessary. The IV:PO conversion is 1:1.

iv. Tapering doses
   - Tapering schedule varies based on protocol and institutional standards. Day of taper initiation and duration of therapy varies from center to center.
   - General rules
     • Related donor nonmyeloablative transplants: Stop MMF on day +28.
     • Unrelated donor nonmyeloablative transplants: Decrease to BID dosing on day +29 with the goal of discontinuing therapy on day +56.

c. Monitoring/adverse effects
   i. Cardiovascular
      - Hypertension
      - Edema
   ii. Gastrointestinal
      - Diarrhea
      - Nausea/vomiting
   iii. Infection
      - Mycophenolate has been shown to be an independent risk factor for development of CMV infections.
      - Preemptive treatment of positive CMV antigenemia is required to prevent active CMV infection.

5. Sirolimus
   a. Mechanism of action/place in therapy

     i. Inhibits both T and B lymphocyte proliferation by binding to FK-binding protein 12, resulting in a complex that directly affects the function of mTOR, an enzyme responsible for growth of cells in the G phase.

    ii. Thought to have synergy with calcineurin inhibitors, sirolimus is used in conjunction with tacrolimus ± methotrexate for myeloablative and non-myeloablative transplants.

b. Dose and administration

    i. Myeloablative and nonmyeloablative transplants

      – Load with 12 mg PO ×1 beginning day –3 followed by 4 mg PO daily

      – If BSA is <1.5 m^2, load with 6 mg/m^2 PO ×1 followed by 2 mg/m^2 PO daily

    ii. Other information

      – There is no IV formulation.

      – Consistently taken medication with or without meals will help with monitoring of levels and dose adjustments.

      – Repeat dose if patient vomits within 15 min of administration. However, $t_{1/2}$ life is very long (60 h), and missing a dose is not likely to affect serum levels.

c. Monitoring

    i. Goal trough concentration is 3–12 ng/mL

    ii. Checking Levels

      – Levels are to be checked no sooner than 5 days following a change in dose or schedule.

      – Routine monitoring of levels should occur once a week.

d. Dose adjustments

    i. Dose adjust for drug interactions with CYP 3A4 Inhibitors such as amiodarone, azole antifungals, calcium channel blockers, nicardipine, macrolide antibiotics, protease inhibitors, and some tyrosine kinase inhibitors.

      – Depending on the strength of azole antifungal as an inhibitor, sirolimus doses may need to be reduced by as much as 60% when given concomitantly with the azole.

      – Concomitant administration with voriconazole may require sirolimus to taken every other day. Inhibition of 3A4 in the gut wall by voriconazole can result in a 100-fold increase in sirolimus concentration.

    ii. Adjust dose for drug interactions with CYP 3A4 inducers such as carbamazepine, phenobarbital, phenytoin, rifabutin, rifampin.

  e. Common toxicities

    i. Cardiovascular
- Hypertension
- Edema

    ii. Pulmonary
- Epistaxis
- Interstitial pneumonitis

    iii. Headache

    iv. Hypercholesterolemia/hypertriglyceridemia

    v. Mild, reversible, leukopenia/anemia/thrombocytopenia with chronic use

    vi. Sirolimus may potentiate transplant-associated thrombotic microangiopathy (TATMA) when given in conjunction with calcineurin inhibitors.

    vii. Arthralgia

    viii. Hypokalemia

6. Antithymocyte immune globulin (ATG)

  a. Mechanism of action/place in therapy

    i. Polyclonal immune globulin preparations created by immunizing either rabbits or horses with human thymocytes or rabbits with the T-lymphoblastic cell line Jurkat (ATG-Fresenius [non-US availability]).

    ii. Used for prevention of GVHD in myeloablative and nonmyeloablative transplants.

  b. Dose and administration

    i. Rabbit ATG: 3–3.75 mg/kg/dose given for 2–5 days pre-transplant for a total of 7.5–15 mg/kg/regimen

    ii. Equine ATG: 10–40 mg/kg/dose often given for 3–4 days pre-transplant (days –5 or −4 through day −2) for a total of 30–160 mg/kg/regimen.

    iii. Premedicate with acetaminophen 650 mg PO, diphenhydramine 50 mg PO/IV, and dexamethasone 20 mg IV 1 h prior to each dose.

    iv. Infuse through central line over a minimum of 6 h on first infusion and 4 h on consecutive infusions.

    v. Requires test dose of 0.1 mL of 1:1,000 dilution intradermally with control of NS 0.1 mL intradermally to the contralateral forearm.
- Observation required every 15 min.

- A positive skin test is a wheal ≥10 mm in diameter.
- Positive skin test, itching, or marked local swelling should invoke reconsideration for further treatment including increasing steroid premeds, or if reaction is severe, holding administration of medication.

  c. Monitoring/adverse effects
   i. Anaphylaxis
      - Have emergency medications at bedside including epinephrine 1:1000 SQ (usual dose 0.3 mg), diphenhydramine 50 mg IV, hydrocortisone 100 mg IV
   ii. Fevers/chills
   iii. Rash
   iv. Joint pain/weakness (serum sickness)
   v. Renal impairment
   vi. Leukopenia/thrombocytopenia

References

Alyea, E.P., Li, S., Kim, H.T., Cutler, C., Ho, V., Soiffer, R.J., et al. (2008). Sirolimus, tacrolimus, and low-dose methotrexate as graft-versus-host disease prophylaxis in related and unrelated donor reduced-intensity conditioning allogeneic peripheral blood stem cell transplantation. *Biol Blood Marrow Transplant*, 14: 920–926.

Ancın, I., Ferra, C., Gallardo, D., Peris, J., Berlanga, J., Gonzalez, J.R., Virgili, N., et al. (2001). Do corticosteroids add any benefit to standard GVHD prophylaxis in allogeneic BMT? *Bone Marrow Transplant*, 28:39–45.

Antin, J.H., Kim, H.T., Cutler, C., Ho, V.T., Lee, S.J., Miklos, D.B., et al. (2003). Sirolimus, tacrolimus, and low-dose methotrexate for graft-versus-host disease prophylaxis in mismatched related donor or unrelated donor transplantation. *Blood*, 102:1601–1605.

Bacigalupo, A., Lamparelli, T., Bruzzi, P., Guidi, S., Alessandrino, P.E., di Bartolomeo, P., et al. (2001). Antithymocyte globulin for graft versus-host disease prophylaxis in transplants from unrelated donors: 2 randomized studies from Gruppo Italiano Trapianti Midollo Osseo (GITMO). *Blood*, 98:2942–2947.

Bensinger, W. (2006). Individual patient data meta-analysis of allogeneic peripheral blood stem cell transplant vs bone marrow transplant in the management of hematological malignancies: Indirect assessment of the effect of day 11 methotrexate administration. *Bone Marrow Transplant*, 38:539–546.

Bolwell, B., Sobecks, R., Pohlman, B., Andresen, S., Rybicki, L., Kuczkowski, E., et al. (2004). A prospective randomized trial comparing cyclosporine and short course methotrexate with cyclosporine and mycophenolate mofetil for GVHD prophylaxis in myeloablative allogeneic bone marrow transplantation. *Bone Marrow Transplant*, 34:621–625.

Bonifazi, F., Bandini, G., Rondelli, D., Falcioni, S., Stanzani, M., Bontadini, A., et al. (2003). Reduced incidence of GVHD without increase in relapse with low-dose rabbit ATG in the preparative regimen for unrelated bone marrow transplants in CML. *Bone Marrow Transplant*, 32:237–242.

Chao, N.J., Snyder, D.S., Jain, M., Wong, R.M., Niland, J.C., Negrin, R.S., et al. (2000). Equivalence of 2 effective graft-versus-host disease prophylaxis regimens: Results of a prospective double-blind randomized trial. *Biol Blood Marrow Transplant*, 6:254–61.

Cutler, C., Antin, J.H. (2004). Sirolimus for GVHD prophylaxis in allogeneic stem cell transplantation. *Bone Marrow Transplant*, 34: 471–476.

Cutler, C., Li, S., Ho, V.T., Koreth, J., Alyea, E., Soiffer, R.J., et al. (2007) Extended follow-up of methotrexate-free immunosuppression using sirolimus and tacrolimus in related and unrelated donor peripheral blood stem cell transplantation. *Blood*, 109: 3108–3114.

Deeg, H.J., Lin, D., Leisenring, W., Boeckh, M., Anasetti, C., Appelbaum, F.R., et al. (1997). Cyclosporine or cyclosporine plus methylprednisolone for prophylaxis of graft-versus-host disease: A prospective, randomized trial. *Blood*, 89:3880–3887.

Finke, J., Schmoor, C., Lang, H., Potthoff, K., Bertz, H. (2003) Matched and mismatched allogeneic stem-cell transplantation from unrelated donors using combined graft-versus-host disease prophylaxis including rabbit anti-T lymphocyte globulin. *J Clin Oncol*, 21: 506–513.

Hambach, L., Stadler, M., Dammann, E., Ganser, A., Hertenstein B. (2002). Increased risk of complicated CMV infection with the use of mycophenolate mofetil in allogeneic stem cell transplantation. *Bone Marrow Transplant*, 29:903–906.

Hiraoka, A., Ohashi, Y., Okamoto, S., Moriyama, Y., Nagao, T., Kodera, Y., et al. (2001). Phase III study comparing tacrolimus (FK506) with cyclosporine for graft-versus-host disease prophylaxis after allogeneic bone marrow transplantation. *Bone Marrow Transplant*, 28:181–185.

Ho, V.T., Aldridge, J., Kim, H.T., Cutler, C., Koreth, J., Armand, P., et al. (2009). Comparison of tacrolimus and sirolimus (Tac/Sir) versus tacrolimus, sirolimus, and mini-methotrexate (Tac/Sir/MTX) as acute graft-versus-host disease prophylaxis after reduced-intensity conditioning allogeneic peripheral blood stem cell transplantation. *Biol Blood Marrow Transplant*, 15:844–850.

Hoyt, R., Ritchie, D.S., Roberts, A.W., MacGregor, L., Curtis, D.J., Szer, J., et al. (2008). Cyclosporine, methotrexate and prednisolone for graft-versus-host disease prophylaxis in allogeneic peripheral blood progenitor cell transplants. *Bone Marrow Transplant*, 41: 651–658.

Kansu, E., Gooley, T., Flowers, M.E., Anasetti, C., Deeg, H.J., Nash, R.A., et al. (2001). Administration of cyclosporine for 24 months compared with 6 months for prevention of chronic graft-versus-host disease: A prospective randomized clinical trial. *Blood*, 98: 3868–3870.

Kasper, C., Sayer, H.G., Mugge, L.O., Schilling, K., Scholl, S., Issa, M.C., et al. (2004). Combined standard graft versus-host disease (GvHD) prophylaxis with mycophenolate mofetil (MMF) in allogeneic peripheral blood stem cell transplantation from unrelated donors. *Bone Marrow Transplant*, 33:65–69.

Kiehl, M.G., Shipkova, M., Basara, N., Blau, W.I., Fauser, A.A. (2000). New strategies in GVHD prophylaxis. *Bone Marrow Transplant*, 25 (Suppl 2), S16–S19.

Mohty, M., de Lavallade, H., Faucher,C., Bilger, K., Vey, N., Stoppa, A.M., et al. (2004) Mycophenolate mofetil and cyclosporine for graft-versus-host disease prophylaxis following reduced intensity conditioning allogeneic stem cell transplantation. *Bone Marrow Transplant*, 34:527–530.

Nash, R.A., Antin, J.H., Karanes, C., Fay, J.W., Avalos, B.R., Yeager, A.M., et al. (2000). Phase 3 study comparing methotrexate and tacrolimus with methotrexate and cyclosporine for prophylaxis of acute graft-versus-host disease after marrow transplantation from unrelated donors. *Blood*, 96:2062–2068.

Nash, R.A., Johnston, L., Parker, P., McCune, J.S., Storer, B., Slattery, J.T., et al. (2005). A phase I/II study of mycophenolate mofetil in combination with cyclosporine for prophylaxis of acute graft-versus-host disease after myeloablative conditioning and allogeneic hematopoietic cell transplantation. *Biol Blood Marrow Transplant*, 11:495–505.

Neumann, F., Graef, T., Tapprich, C., Vaupel, M., Steidl, U., Germing, U., et al. (2005). Cyclosporine A and mycophenolate mofetil vs cyclosporine A and methotrexate for graft-versus-host disease prophylaxis after stem cell transplantation from HLA-identical siblings. *Bone Marrow Transplant*, 35:1089–1093.

Niederwieser, D., Maris, M., Shizuru, J.A., Petersdorf, E., te Hegenbart, U., Sandmaier, B.M., et al. (2003). Low dose total body irradiation (TBI) and fludarabine followed by hematopoietic cell transplantation (HCT) from HLA-matched or mismatched unrelated donors and postgrafting immunosuppression with cyclosporine and mycophenolate mofetil (MMF) can induce durable complete chimerism and sustained remissions in patients with hematological diseases. *Blood*, 101:1620–1629.

Nieto, Y., Patton, N., Hawkins, T., Spearing, R., Bearman, S.I., Jones, R.B., et al. (2006). Tacrolimus and mycophenolate mofetil after nonmyeloablative matched-sibling donor allogeneic stem-cell transplantations conditioned with fludarabine and low-dose total body irradiation. *Biol Blood Marrow Transplant*, 12:217–225.

Ogawa, N., Kanda, Y., Matsubara, M., Asano, Y., Nakagawa, M., Sakata-Yanagimoto, M., et al. (2004). Increased incidence of acute graft-versus-host disease with the continuous infusion of cyclosporine A compared to twice-daily infusion. *Bone Marrow Transplant*, 33: 549–552.

Perez-Simon, J.A., Martino, R., Caballero, D., Valcarcel, D., Rebollo, N., de la Camara, R., et al. (2008). Reduced intensity conditioning allogeneic transplantation from unrelated donors: Evaluation of mycophenolate mofetil plus cyclosporin A as graft-versus-host disease prophylaxis. *Biol Blood Marrow Transplant*, 14: 664–671.

Przepiorka, D., Nash, R.A., Wingard, J.R., Zhu, J., Maher, R.M., Fitzsimmons, W.E., et al. (1999). Relationship of tacrolimus whole blood levels to efficacy and safety outcomes after unrelated donor marrow transplantation. *Biol Blood Marrow Transplant*, 5:94–97.

Punnett, A., Sung, L., Price, V., Das, P., Diezi, M., Doyle, J., et al. (2007). Achievement of target cyclosporine concentrations as a predictor of severe acute graft versus host disease in children undergoing hematopoietic stem cell transplantation and receiving cyclosporine and methotrexate prophylaxis. *Ther Drug Monit*, 29:750–757.

Quellmann, S., Schwarzer, G., Hübel, K., Greb, A., Engert, A., Bohlius, J. (2008). Corticosteroids for preventing graft versus-host disease after allogeneic myeloablative stem cell transplantation. *Cochrane Database Syst Rev*, (3).

Ratanatharathorn, V., Nash, R.A., Przepiorka, D., Devine, S.M., Klein, J.L., Weisdorf, D., et al. (1998). Phase III study comparing methotrexate and tacrolimus (prograf, FK506) with methotrexate and cyclosporine for graft-versus-host disease prophylaxis after HLA-identical sibling bone marrow transplantation. *Blood*, 92:2303–2314.

Rodriguez, R., Parker, P., Nademanee, A., Smith, D., O'Donnell, M.R., Stein, A., et al. (2004). Cyclosporine and mycophenolate mofetil prophylaxis with fludarabine and melphalan conditioning for unrelated donor transplantation: A prospective study of 22 patients with hematologic malignancies. *Bone Marrow Transplant*, 33: 1123–1129.

Ruutu, T., Volin, L., Parkkali, T., Juvonen, E., Elonen, E. (2000). Cyclosporine, methotrexate, and methylprednisolone compared with cyclosporine and methotrexate for the prevention of graft-versus-host disease in bone marrow transplantation from HLA-identical sibling donor: A prospective randomized study. *Blood*, 96:2391–2398.

Sabry, W., Le Blanc, R., Labbe, A.C., Sauvageau, G., Couban, S., Kiss, T., et al. (2009). Graft-versus-host disease prophylaxis with tacrolimus and mycophenolate mofetil in HLA-matched nonmyeloablative transplant recipients is associated with very low incidence of GVHD and nonrelapse mortality. *Biol Blood Marrow Transplant*, 15:919–929.

Uberti, J.P., Ayash, L., Braun, T., Reynolds, C., Silver, S., Ratanatharathorn, V. (2004). Tacrolimus as monotherapy or combined with minidose methotrexate for graft-versus-host disease prophylaxis after allogeneic peripheral blood stem cell transplantation: Long-term outcomes. *Bone Marrow Transplant*, 34:425–431.

Wingard, J.R., Nash, R.A., Przepiorka, D., Klein, J.L., Weisdorf, D.J., Fay, J.W., et al. (1998). Relationship of tacrolimus (FK506) whole blood concentrations and efficacy and safety after HLA identical sibling bone marrow transplantation *Biol Blood and Marrow Transplant*, 4:157–163.

Yanik, G., Levine, J.E., Ratanatharathorn, V., Dunn, R., Ferrara, J., Hutchinson, R.J. (2000). Tacrolimus (FK506) and methotrexate as prophylaxis for acute graft versus-host disease in pediatric allogeneic stem cell transplantation. *Bone Marrow Transplant*, 26: 161–167.

Zander, A.R., Kroger, N., Schleuning, M., Finke, J., Zabelina, T., Beelen, D., et al. (2003). ATG as part of the conditioning regimen reduces transplant-related mortality (TRM) and improves overall survival after unrelated stem cell transplantation in patients with chronic myelogenous leukemia (CML). *Bone Marrow Transplant*, 32: 355–361.

CHAPTER 10
Transfusion Medicine

James Gajewski and Susan Slater

The unique transfusion needs of a hematopoietic stem cell transplant (HSCT) patient require collaboration between the Clinical Transplant and Transfusion Medicine services. Successful interaction is essential to the optimal management of HSCT patients with the goals of reducing the risk of alloimmunization, infection transmission, and avoiding potential medical errors.

10.1 PRE-TRANSPLANT CONSIDERATIONS

1. All transplant candidates should receive leukocyte reduced red blood cell and platelet products
   a. Decreases the incidence of alloimmunization to HLA antigens
      i. Positive lymphocytotoxic and flow cytometric cross-match studies are associated with increased risk of primary graft failure and graft rejection
   b. Reduces the risk of transfusion-associated CMV transmission
      i. All patients should have a pre-transplant assessment of CMV exposure as determined by serum anti-CMV titers
      ii. Leukofiltration has been shown in randomized trials to be effective at decreasing donor-derived CMV transmission
      iii. Utilization of CMV negative blood products is the best way to prevent CMV transmission in CMV-negative patients receiving a product from a CMV-negative HSC donor

R.T. Maziarz, S. Slater (eds.), *Blood and Marrow Transplant Handbook*, DOI 10.1007/978-1-4419-7506-5_10, © Springer Science+Business Media, LLC 2011

2. All blood products should also be irradiated to a dose of 1,500–2,500 cGy
   a. Reduces the incidence of transfusion-associated graft-versus-host disease (TA-GvHD) secondary to introduction of donor lymphocytes
      i. Clinical symptoms of TA-GvHD occur between 4 and 30 days post-transplant and may include:
         – Fever
         – Macular papular rash
         – Bloody diarrhea
         – Pancytopenia
      ii. Uncommon syndrome but with mortality rate ~88%
   b. There are no data available to verify lifetime need for irradiated blood products; however, most centers recommend this safety maneuver as standard practice as there are no reliable tests to measure complete immunologic reconstitution
   c. HSC donors should also receive irradiated blood products during stem cell collection to reduce the theoretical transmission risk of TA-GvHD associated with transfusions of non-irradiated blood products.
3. Special concerns for patient with aplastic anemia
   a. Multiply transfused aplastic anemia patients have increased rates of graft rejection resulting in decreased rates of overall survival
   b. The number of blood transfusions should be minimized whenever possible, and platelet products should be single-donor products to reduce the number of donor exposures
   c. Use of blood components from family members who are potential donors should be discouraged to avoid immunologically sensitizing the recipient to the potential donor's minor histocompatibility antigens and HLA if a mismatched relative is the only donor option.

10.2 PERI-TRANSPLANT CONSIDERATIONS

1. Selection of a donor is based on HLA matching criteria; however, occasionally two or more donors are equal from an HLA matching perspective. In that case, donor selection will be influenced by:
   a. ABO Rh matching
   b. CMV status matching

    c. Donor age

       i. Increased blood or marrow stem cell harvest risks to older donors

      ii. Concomitant health issues and comorbid clinical conditions in donors

     iii. Younger donor age has been associated with better survival outcomes within similar HLA-matched donor recipient paired populations

    d. Donor/recipient size disparity is often an issue when donors are younger than recipients

       i. Umbilical cord blood

      ii. Haplo-identical donors

2. Major ABO incompatibility

    a. This circumstance exists when the recipient's plasma has anti-donor RBC antibodies (i.e., recipient is blood group O [absence of A, B substances], donor is blood group A or B or AB)

    b. During donor PBSC apheresis collection, hematocrit should be kept to <2% to minimize exposure to incompatible RBC volume

    c. HSC bone marrow product requires RBC-depletion by one of the following methods:

       i. Hetastarch separation

      ii. Mononuclear cell separation by machine centrifugation

     iii. Chemical separation via density gradient separation

     iv. Important to double-check ABO-Rh typing prior to infusion and confirm correct processing has been done. If reaction occurs, stop infusion, recheck typing and processing and, if correct, then an immediate density gradient mononuclear cell preparation is required

3. Minor ABO incompatibility

    a. This circumstance exists when the donor's plasma is incompatible with the recipient's RBCs (i.e., donor is blood group O, recipient is blood group A or B or AB)

    b. Bone marrow products may require plasma reduction if donor anti-recipient titer is high

       i. To decrease risk, many centers will plasma-deplete all minor ABO-incompatible products

      ii. Peripheral blood stem cell products are already plasma and RBC reduced, but are easily further plasma depleted.

iii. There is always concern for minor RBC antibodies not detectable by crossmatch. In these instances, the infusion should be stopped immediately and donor/recipient identity, crossmatch, and antibody screens reviewed. If no error is identified, an immediate density gradient, mononuclear cell separation is required

4. Major-minor ABO incompatibility: mononuclear cell concentration or density gradient mononuclear separation is required
5. Due to major and minor ABO incompatibility between donors and recipients, guidelines for transfusion of blood products have been established to decrease the risk of complications (see Table 10.1).
6. Exact transfusion thresholds have not been defined; however, these will be influenced by comorbid conditions and transplant complications.

TABLE 10.1. Guidelines for selecting ABO group for erythrocyte and platelet-containing components for patients undergoing HSCT

Recipient ABO group	Donor ABO group	Transfuse RBCs	Transfuse platelets/plasma products[a]
A	B	O	AB
A	O	O	A
A	AB	O	AB
B	A	O	AB
B	O	O	B
B	AB	O	AB
O	A	O	A
O	B	O	B
O	AB	O	AB
AB	A	O	AB
AB	B	O	AB
AB	O	O	AB
Rh positive	Rh negative	Rh negative	Rh negative[b]
Rh negative	Rh positive	Rh positive	Rh pos/neg

[a] First choice for platelet transfusions. If first choice is unavailable, use any ABO group for platelet support
[b] Rh-negative platelets first choice. If only Rh-positive platelets available, consult Transfusion service for Rh immunoglobulin dosing

a. Conventional threshold for platelet transfusions is a platelet count of $\leq$10,000/mm^3, following recommendations for acute leukemia patients having chemotherapy-induced aplasia.

   i. Platelet consumption is not usually dependent on transfusion parameters, but rather on whether the patient has an active bleeding diathesis. Therefore, the patient's clinical situation should be considered when establishing platelet transfusion parameters

   ii. For patients who do not demonstrate an incremental increase to transfused platelet products as assessed by a 15–30 min post-platelet count, initiation of a platelet-refractory work-up should be initiated to determine the extent of alloimmunization

b. Conventional threshold for PRBC transfusions is Hgb $\leq$8 g/dL

   i. Patients with coronary artery disease or ischemic heart disease may require higher transfusion thresholds.

10.3 DAY 0 TRANSPLANT INFUSION CONSIDERATIONS

1. Standard practice for all patients includes pre-medication with acetaminophen 650 mg po, diphenhydramine 25–50 mg IV/po, and IV steroids (hydrocortisone 100 mg IV or equivalent) prior to infusion of both autologous and allogeneic stem cell products, with institution specific variations. The donor–recipient HLA disparity and whether ex vivo or in vivo T-cell depletion are additional determinants of prophylaxis needs.

   a. Emergency medications should be at the bedside during stem cell infusion including:

      i. Acetaminophen

      ii. Diphenhydramine IV

      iii. Hydrocortisone IV (or equivalent)

      iv. Epinephrine (1:1,000)

      v. Dopamine (or alternate vasopressor)

2. Marrow

   a. Volume overload can be seen on occasion with transfusion of 2–3 units PRBC equivalent infusion; diuresis may be needed

   b. Fat emboli syndrome has been reported in the past, but less in the modern era with in-line filters

    c. Bone emboli are potential risks if product is not filtered

    d. Anaphylaxis is usually due to incompatibility from major or minor RBC cell surface antigens, but sometimes also from additives used in cell processing

3. PBSCs

    a. Anaphylaxis is usually due to incompatibility from major or minor RBC cell surface antigens, but sometimes also from additives used in cell processing

    b. Infusion-related toxicities may include hypertension, hypotension, fever, cough, nausea, vomiting, flushing

4. Cryopreserved product infusion

    a. Cold cardioplegia

    b. Rate of infusion will influence toxicity, i.e., hypotension, systemic symptoms

    c. Number of granulocytes in the product influences risk of DMSO toxicity

    d. DMSO is very lipid-soluble, so during infusion, as thawed cryopreserved product reaches the pulmonary vascular bed, transalveolar diffusion occurs and patient may experience dysphoric sensations of taste, throat constriction, cough

    e. Neurologic toxicity has also been reported

    f. DMSO removal has not adversely affected outcomes

5. Transplant-associated hemolysis

    a. There is always a risk of immediate hemolysis due to recipient antidonor antibodies.

        i. This occasionally occurs in the autologous transplant setting and is typically an allergic reaction to DMSO used in the cryopreservation process.

            – With the cryopreservation process, red cells often fracture; interaction between these red cells and circulating red cells can mimic a transfusion reaction even with autologous infusions

            – Some centers routinely wash DMSO from cryopreserved products prior to infusion

            – Always important to recheck with source documents at infusion, donor–recipient product identity, confirm donor–recipient HLA type, donor–recipient HLA type, and RBC/plasma processing performed. If all correct pathways followed, then in allogeneic setting, an immediate mononuclear separation should be performed

10.4 POST-TRANSPLANT CONSIDERATIONS

1. Immune hemolysis
   a. Hemolysis immediately post-transplant results from recipient-derived anti-erythrocyte antibodies; delayed hemolysis is likely due to donor ABO antibodies
   b. Passenger lymphocyte syndrome
      i. Typically involves ABO incompatibility and antibody production by the donor's lymphocytes in the HSC product.
      ii. Risk factors
         – PBSC product > marrow
         – Use of cyclosporine without methotrexate for GvHD prophylaxis
         – Reduced-intensity preparative regimen
      iii. Clinical management focuses on monitoring for signs of acute hemolysis and transfusing PRBCs at a rate to maintain a stable hematocrit.
   c. Pure red cell aplasia
      i. May result after major ABO-mismatched HSCT transplants
         – Recipients lymphocytes and/or plasma plasma cells persist after completion of the conditioning regimen and produce antibodies to donor-derived erythrocytes, resulting in destruction of erythroid precursors and anemia.
      ii. Can occur either early or late (>100 days) post-transplant
      iii. Diagnosis requires persistence of reticulocytopenia for more than 60 days post-transplant and absence of erythrocytes in the marrow.
      iv. DDx includes parvovirus B-19
         – Check parvovirus IgM or parvovirus DNA
      v. Treatment
         – Plasma exchange to remove hemagluttinins although this has not been shown to be effective due to its short effect and rapid rebound
         – Decrease immune suppression to induce a graft-versus-host effect.
   d. Autoimmune hemolytic anemia (AIHA)
      i. Occasionally occurs post-HSCT with no specific time-frame
      ii. Diagnosis should be considered for a positive direct Coombs

iii. Study results may show a warm type (IgG) panagglutinin, cold type (IgM) agglutinin, or an antibody with relative serologic specificity for other blood-group antigens.

iv. Late AIHA is associated with poor survival

v. More common in T-cell-depleted grafts

vi. Usually associated with either T-cell dysregulation or viral infection, but can often be an early sign of impending relapse.

2. Engraftment syndrome

  a. Typically presents with fever and hypoxia which coincide with WBC recovery

  b. May progress to diffuse-alveolar hemorrhage (see Chapter 19)

  c. High-dose steroids are used for initial therapy; however, an increased platelet transfusion parameter may be required for patients who develop DAH

    i. Consider recombinant factor VIIa or aminocaproic acid for persistent bleeding

3. Transfer back to community setting

It is important to advise local medical providers of correct transfusion practice. These providers and local transfusion services are not always familiar with ABO type changes that occur following allogeneic HSCT or the need for irradiated blood products in all transplant recipients. Transfer of care letters should consider including information on appropriate transfusion practice.

Patients should also be made aware of their unique transfusion needs. They should be alerted to carry appropriate identification, e.g., Med alert bracelets alerting care providers in case the patient is rendered unconscious or unable to provide medical history.

References

Boeckh, M., Nichols, W., Papanicolaou, G., Rubin, R., Wingard, J., Zaia, J. (2003). Cytomegalovirus in hematopoietic stem cell transplants: Current status, known challenges, and future strategies. *Bio Blood Marrow Transplant*, 9:543–558.

Gajewski, J., Petz, L., Calhoun, L., et. al. (1992). Hemolysis of transfused group O red blood cells in minor ABO-incompatible unrelated-donor bone marrow transplants in patients receiving cyclosporine without posttransplant methotrexate. *Blood*, 79:3076–3085.

Gajewski, J., Johnson, V., Sandler, G., Sayegh, A., Klumpp, T. (2008). A review of transfusion practice before, during, and after hematopoietic progenitor cell transplantation. *Blood*, 112:3036–3047.

Klumpp, T. (1991). Immunohematologic complications of bone marrow transplantation. *Bone Marrow Transplant*, 8:159–170.

Lapierre, V., Mahé, C., Aupérin, A., et. al. (2005). Platelet transfusion containing ABO-incompatible plasma and hepatic veno-occlusive disease after hematopoietic transplantation in young children. *Transplant*, 80:314–319.

LaRoche, V., Eastlund, D., McCullough, J. (2004). Review: Immunohematologic aspects of allogeneic hematopoietic progenitor cell transplantation. *Immunohematology*, 20:217–225.

Nevo, S., Fuller, A., Zahurak, M., Hartley, E., Borinsky, M., Volgesang, G. (2007). Profound thrombocytopenia and survival of hematopoietic stem cell transplant patients without clinically significant bleeding, using prophylactic platelet transfusion triggers of 10×10^9 or 20×10^9/L. *Transfusion*, 49:1700–1709.

Petz LD. (1987). Immunohematologic problems associated with bone marrow transplantation. *Transfusion Med Rev*, 1:85–100.

Pihusch, M. (2004). Bleeding complications after hematopoietic stem cell transplantation. *Semin Hematol*, 41(Supp 1):93–100.

Stroncek, D., McCullough, J. (1997). Policies and procedures for the establishment of an allogeneic blood stem cell collection program. *Transfus Med*, 7:77–87.

Worel, N., Grenix, H., Keil, F., et al. (2002). Severe immune hemolysis after minor ABO-mismatched allogeneic peripheral blood progenitor cell transplantation occurs more frequently after nonmyeloablative than myeloablative conditioning. *Transfusion*, 42:1293–1301.

CHAPTER 11
Antithrombotic Guidelines

Thomas DeLoughery

Patients receiving stem cell transplantation with specialized needs regarding antithrombotic therapy can fall into two basic groups: those who are on pre-transplant therapy and those who develop thrombosis during the course of the procedure. See Table 11.1 for a summary of management guidelines.

11.1 PATIENTS ON ANTITHROMBOTIC THERAPY

1. Antiplatelet therapy
   a. Primary prevention
      i. A significant portion of the population is on aspirin or other antiplatelet agents.
      ii. In recent years, the use of these drugs for primary prevention of first myocardial infarction or stroke has become controversial.
      iii. The absolute reduction in events is very small and almost balanced by the increase risk in bleeding. Therefore, for a transplant patient taking antiplatelet agents for this indication, the most reasonable procedure would be to stop the medication.
   b. Secondary prevention
      i. The benefits of antiplatelet therapy are more robust with patients seeing a 22% reduction in vascular events for secondary prevention of strokes or myocardial infarctions.
      ii. A reasonable strategy would be to stop the drug when conditioning starts and then resume when platelets have recovered over 50,000/μL.

R.T. Maziarz, S. Slater (eds.), *Blood and Marrow Transplant Handbook*, DOI 10.1007/978-1-4419-7506-5_11, © Springer Science+Business Media, LLC 2011

TABLE 11.1. Management guidelines

Aspirin	
• Primary prevention	Stop
• Secondary prevention	Stop during conditioning, resume when platelets >50,000
Coronary stent	
• Bare metal	Combined therapy (ASA + thienopyridine) 4 weeks, then ASA thereafter. Continue ASA until platelet count <20,000, then resume when >20,000
• Drug eluting	If possible, delay transplant until 1 year after stent placement. If unable, combined therapy throughout transplant. After 1 year, continue ASA until platelet count <20,000 then resuming when >20,000
Atrial fibrillation	
• CHADS2 0–2	Stop ASA during conditioning, resume when platelets >50,000
• CHADS2 > 2	Therapeutic LMWH until platelets <50,000, prophylactic dosing when platelets 20–50,000
Mechanical heart valve	Therapeutic LMWH until platelets <50,000, prophylactic doses 20–50,000
Acute events	
• Catheter thrombosis	Remove catheter, consider anticoagulation if symptomatic and platelets >50,000
• Distal thrombosis	Follow up scans in 3 days, then weekly
• Proximal thrombosis and PE	Therapeutic LMWH if platelets >50,000, prophylactic doses 20–50,000, IVC filter if platelets <20,000
Acute coronary syndrome	ASA for all patients regardless of platelet count
	Individual therapy for patient per cardiology recommendations

iii. Patients with a history of myocardial infarction, stroke, or vascular disease, but not previously on therapy, should be started on aspirin 81 mg daily (or clopidogrel 75 mg po daily if aspirin intolerant) when platelets have recovered.
c. Patients with coronary stents
    i. Management of patients with coronary stents is difficult because stopping antiplatelet therapy is strongly

associated with stent thrombosis, which can be fatal in up to 50% of patients.

ii. The risk is most extreme for bare metal stents for 4 weeks after placement and with drug-eluting stents (DES) up to 1 year after placement. During this period, even stopping just clopidogrel is associated with adverse outcomes.

iii. For a patient with a DES stent who needs transplantation during the "at-risk" period, it may be prudent to continue dual antiplatelet therapy throughout the phase of thrombocytopenia unless bleeding develops.

iv. If possible, consideration should be given to delaying transplant until a year after DES placement, and consultation with cardiology is mandatory before transplant.

v. For patients with stents outside the high-risk period, continuing aspirin until the platelet count is under 20,000/μL and then resuming when greater than 20,000/μL can be considered.

11.2 ANTITHROMBOTIC THERAPY

1. Choice of therapy during transplantation

   a. Although warfarin (Coumadin®) is the antithrombotic agent of choice for most patients, many of its properties make it undesirable for the transplant patient.

      i. Warfarin requires close monitoring, has many drug–drug and food interactions, level of anticoagulation is dependent on vitamin K intake, and the half-life is 36 h, making it impractical to quickly start and stop if for changes in clinical condition.

   b. The most practical antithrombotic agents for transplantation are the low molecular weight heparins (LMWH – see Table 11.2). The lack of interactions and the relatively short half-life ($\sim$ 4 h) simplifies their use in this setting. The one caution is that all these agents are renally cleared so they need to be closely monitored if used in patients with severe renal insufficiency.

   c. There is no clear guidance on what platelet count level is the threshold for anticoagulation, but most experts would recommend no full dose anticoagulation below a platelet count of 50,000/μL and no prophylactic anticoagulation below a platelet count of 20,000/μL.

TABLE 11.2. Low molecular weight heparins

Drug	Prophylactic dosing	Therapeutic dosing	Pediatric dosing
Daltaparin	2500 units/day	100 units/kg q 12 h	
Enoxaparin	40 mg/day	1 mg/kg q 12 h or 1.5 mg/kg/day in low-risk patients	<5 kg: 1.5 mg/kg q 12 h >5 kg: 1 mg/kg q 12 h
Tinzaparin	3500 units/day	175 units/day	

    d. In theory, one can give platelet transfusions to patients to try to keep the platelets above these thresholds, but in practice this is difficult and is associated with excess bleeding.

2. Atrial fibrillation

    a. The leading indication for warfarin in older patients is stroke prevention from atrial fibrillation.

       i. It is estimated that 15% of all strokes can be attributed to atrial fibrillation. Warfarin reduced the stroke rate from 5% per year to 1%.

      ii. While warfarin benefits most patients, patients who previously have had strokes are at higher risk of stroke and appear to benefit the most from anticoagulation.

    b. Data now exist to risk-stratify patients and help to choose between warfarin and aspirin therapy.

       i. Clinically, the most useful prediction rule appears to be the CHADS2 rule, with one point being assessed for the presence of congestive heart failure, hypertension, age over 75, diabetes, and two points for history of stroke (see Table 11.3).

      ii. For the average patient, a CHADS2 score of 0–1 would suggest low risk of stroke and aspirin therapy while higher score (≥ 2) support the use of warfarin.

     iii. For individuals with a score ≥ 2 using the CHADS2 classification, lifelong anticoagulation is recommended unless a contraindication emerges.

     iv. For management of a transplant patient with their expected periods of thrombocytopenia, those patients with CHADS2 scores of 0–1 would stop aspirin at a platelet count of 50,000/μL and resume when platelets recover to over that level.

TABLE 11.3. CHADS2 scoring system

CHADS2 score	Yearly risk of stroke	Therapy
0	1.9	Aspirin
1	2.8	Aspirin
2	4.0	Warfarin
3	5.9	Warfarin
4	8.5	Warfarin
5	12.5	Warfarin
6	18.2	Warfarin

One point each for recent heart failure, hypertension, age >75, and diabetes. Two points assigned for history of stroke

  v. Patients with higher CHADS2 scores should be anti-coagulated with LMWH as outlined above in point 1.b in Section 11.2.

3. Mechanical cardiac valves
  a. Patients with mechanical heart valves have high risk for embolization/valve thrombosis, and anticoagulation is strongly recommended.
      i. The estimated risk of thrombosis without anticoagulant ranges from 12 to 30%/year.
     ii. Data support the idea that the newer generation of mechanical valves are less thrombogenic than the older ball-cage valves.
    iii. Even with anticoagulation, the yearly rate of thrombosis ranges from 2.5% with ball-cage to 0.5% with a bileaflet valve.
     iv. For management of a transplant patient with their expected periods of thrombocytopenia, no full-dose anticoagulation below a platelet count of 50,000/μL and no prophylactic anticoagulation below a platelet count of 20,000/μL is recommended.
      v. The daily risk of stroke off anticoagulation is uncertain, but recent data suggest it may be as high as 0.5–1%, and this risk needs to be factored into risk assessment for transplantation.
     vi. For patients perceived to be a very high thrombosis risk (i.e., mitral valve with atrial fibrillation and history of stroke), one may consider platelet threshold of 30,000/μL for therapeutic LMWH; however,

this would be associated with increased risk of bleeding.

   vii. Patients with mechanical aortic valves are at lesser risk of thrombosis than those with mitral valves, and those with atrial fibrillation are at higher risk. However, the rates of embolism and valve thrombosis are still substantial with newer valves, and anticoagulation is still mandatory.

b. Although the risk is lower than mechanical valves, bioprosthetic heart valves still have a definite risk of associated embolization and aspirin therapy is used. For transplant patients with bioprosthetic valves, aspirin should be stopped at a platelet count of 50,000/μL and resumed when platelets recover to over that level.

   i. Patients with bioprosthetic valves with other risk factors such as atrial fibrillation or history of embolic stroke should be anticoagulated with LMWH as outlined above.

4. Deep venous thrombosis

a. The duration of therapy for DVT is determined by both the circumstances of the thrombosis and its location.

   i. Provoked thrombosis (due to surgery, estrogen, trauma, etc.) need only 3 months of anticoagulation, while those below the popliteal vein need at the most 6 weeks.

   ii. Idiopathic thrombosis, especially pulmonary embolism, should be considered for lifelong anticoagulation.

b. The risk of recurrent thrombosis is thought to be highest 6–12 weeks after the event so for most patients, even those requiring long-term anticoagulation, LMWH may be the therapy of choice, as outlined above.

c. Although rare, DVT can complicate transplantations.

   i. Rates are reported to be higher as the patient recovers and are hospitalized later for complications.

   ii. Thrombosis incidences are similar to any general medicine patient (~1% symptomatic and 15% on screening).

   iii. Given the risk of bleeding, intermittent compression stockings should be use for DVT prophylaxis.

   iv. For hospitalized patients who have recovered their platelet counts, LMWH or other pharmacological prophylaxis should be used, especially if for severe infection or other major complications.

11.3 PATIENTS WHO DEVELOP THROMBOSIS

1. Catheter thrombosis
   a. Central venous catheters are essential to many aspects of cancer therapy. The clinically apparent thrombosis incidence for catheters ranges from 5 to 30% and can be as high as 40% with PICCs.
   b. Signs of catheter thrombosis are nonspecific, leading to the finding that incidence of thrombosis is underestimated and can be as high as 50% if screening is performed.
   c. Unlike lower extremity thrombosis, the incidence of PE with upper thrombosis is much less – only 8% vs. 31% in one study.
   d. Prevention of catheter thrombosis is controversial and most likely futile.
      i. Most studies have not shown a benefit to prophylaxis with LMWH or warfarin in preventing thrombosis, and prophylaxis is not warranted in the transplant setting.
   e. Therapy starts with removing the catheter, because this will remove the provoker of the thrombus and is the only clinical step associated with greater recanalization of the vein.
      i. If the patient is not severely thrombocytopenic but symptomatic, one can consider anticoagulation for 4–6 weeks. There are data that one can try to "salvage" the catheter by keeping it in and using anticoagulation, but this was associated with a 4% incidence of serious bleeding in a pilot study.
      ii. Given the low risk of long-term sequela, there is little indication for thrombolytic therapy unless there is massive thrombosis (i.e., SVC syndrome).
   f. Rarely, catheter thrombosis can be a sign of heparin-induced thrombocytopenia since heparin is often used to ensure patency. This diagnosis should be considered if there is massive thrombosis or coincidental thrombosis in other vascular fields.
2. Deep venous thrombosis
   a. If diagnosed during the thrombocytopenic phase, distal thrombosis can just be observed with a Doppler scan 3 days later, and then weekly or sooner if symptoms increase.
   b. For the thrombocytopenic patient with a proximal vein thrombosis or pulmonary embolism, an inferior vena

cava filter should be placed until the patient can be anticoagulated.

   i. Again a platelet threshold of 50,000/µL should be used to start anticoagulation.

   ii. Patient should be anticoagulated for 3 months since these would be considered "provoked thrombosis."

   iii. Given the complex medical regimens these patients are on, long-term LMWH should be used for therapy.

3. Acute coronary syndrome

   a. Modern management of acute coronary syndrome (ACS) involves intense anticoagulation therapy.

   b. The presence of severe thrombocytopenia precludes the use of combined therapy with aspirin, clopidogrel, heparin, and intravenous platelet inhibitors.

      i. However, the use of aspirin is crucial for any patient with an acute coronary syndrome and should be given to any transplant patient with ACS, no matter what the platelet count is.

   c. Further management of the transplant patient with ACS needs to be individual dependent on the stage of transplant they are in and their clinic condition. The Cardiologist and Transplant Provider need to coordinate care thoroughly in the difficult cases.

References

ACCP Guidelines. (2008, Jun). Antithrombotic and thrombolytic therapy, 8th ed. *Chest* 133(Suppl), 67S–968S.

Grines, C.L., Bonow, R.O., Casey, D.E. Jr, Gardner, T.J., Lockhart, P.B., Moliterno, D.J., et al. (2007). Prevention of premature discontinuation of dual antiplatelet therapy in patients with coronary artery stents: A science advisory from the American Heart Association, American College of Cardiology, Society for Cardiovascular Angiography and Interventions, American College of Surgeons, and American Dental Association, with representation from the American College of Physicians. *Circulation*, 115:813–818.

Jones, M.A., Lee, D.Y., Segall, J.A., Landry, G.J., Liem, T.K., Mitchell, E.L., et al. (2010). Characterizing resolution of catheter-associated upper extremity deep venous thrombosis. *J Vasc Surg*, 51:108–113.

CHAPTER 12
Engraftment

Sara Murray

Engraftment after high-dose therapy appears to occur as "overlapping waves" of hematopoiesis. Initial increases in absolute neutrophil counts result from a transferred population of relatively mature committed progenitor cells that are capable of only transient engraftment. Immature multipotent stem cells generate the second phase of neutrophil engraftment. Finally, pluripotent stem cells from the transplanted graft sustain tri-lineage hematopoiesis. Generally, engraftment begins to be observed 10–21 days after the stem cell infusion. Engraftment kinetics can be influenced by a number of factors including the underlying disease, pre-transplant therapy, conditioning regimen, use of cytokines post-transplant, graft quality, and post-transplant complications/events (e.g., GvHD, medications, infections).

Engraftment is defined in a variety of ways by different institutions, but generally has a minimum criteria of (1) an absolute neutrophil count of $\geq 500/mm^3$ for three consecutive days, (2) a platelet count of $\geq 20,000/m^3$ for three consecutive days (and without transfusions for 7 days), and (3) a hematocrit $\geq 25\%$ for at least 20 days (without transfusions).

12.1 AUTOLOGOUS

Initial white blood cell recovery is usually seen 10–14 days after stem cell infusion with platelet and red cell independence occurring at more variable rates. There are no routinely scheduled bone marrow biopsy/aspirate procedures post-autologous PBSC transplant to assess engraftment.

R.T. Maziarz, S. Slater (eds.), *Blood and Marrow Transplant Handbook*, DOI 10.1007/978-1-4419-7506-5_12, © Springer Science+Business Media, LLC 2011

12.2 ALLOGENEIC

Generally, a rise is detected in the peripheral blood granulocyte count in the third week after the stem cell source is infused. Peripheral blood stem cells average 10–14 days until the first evidence of recovery, bone marrow stem cells average 21 days post-infusion. Umbilical cord blood engraftment can even be longer, but can be facilitated by identifying compatible donor cord blood products with higher cell counts. Recovery of platelet production is more delayed, but transfusion independence is usually achieved within 5–7 weeks after transplant and can occur much earlier. Hematocrit and hemoglobin levels are not good indicators of hematopoietic recovery. Patients receiving an ABO incompatible donor stem cell infusion may continue to produce isoagglutinins (host-specific) for months to years. This circumstance may result in diminished reticulocyte activity and delayed red cell transfusion independence.

Neutrophil engraftment time lines are influenced by graft-versus-host disease prophylaxis, with cyclosporine/prednisone showing the shortest engraftment time (10–15 days) and long-course methotrexate/cyclosporine having the longest engraftment time (21–26 days). These observations apply to marrow allografts. Blood stem cell allografts typically recover 2–3 days sooner.

Engraftment following a myeloablative allogeneic PBSC transplant is documented by a bone marrow biopsy often performed between days +60 and +80. Chimerisms are evaluated by either VNTR (same sex donor) or FISH for XY (different sex donor). For nonmyeloablative allogeneic transplants, peripheral chimerisms on both CD3+ (T-cell lymphocytes) and CD 33+ (myeloid lineage) populations are assessed in schedules determined by institutional guidelines. Example of a typical schedule includes assessments at days +28, +56, +84; 6, 12, 18, and 24 months; then annually until 5 years post-transplant. Marrow chimerisms are generally checked at the same intervals as the standard marrow assessments are performed.

12.3 ENGRAFTMENT SYNDROME

There are a constellation of signs and symptoms that may occur during engraftment in patients who undergo autologous blood stem cell or bone marrow transplantation and may cause significant morbidity. The clinical findings of fever, rash, capillary leak, and pulmonary infiltrates can occur as isolated entities or in combination, creating a differential diagnosis dilemma, as the patient is often quite ill. Treatment for "engraftment syndrome" includes diuretics and steroids (1 mg/kg/day), which often result in prompt resolution of symptoms. If the patient is still receiving Filgrastim, this medication should be stopped. The timeline of this syndrome also correlates with the development of diffuse alveolar hemorrhage in both the allogeneic and the autologous patient population.

12.4 FOUNDATION FOR THE ACCREDITATION OF CELLULAR THERAPY (FACT) STANDARDS FOR REVIEW OF ENGRAFTMENT

The major objective of the Foundation for the Accreditation of Cellular Therapy (FACT) is to promote quality medical and laboratory practice in hematopoietic progenitor cell transplantation and other therapies using cellular products. FACT Standards were formed from laboratory standards developed by the International Society for Cellular Therapy (ISCT) and from the clinical and training guidelines developed by the American Society of Blood and Marrow Transplantation (ASBMT). Consensus in medical literature and contributions of experts in the cellular therapy field also led to the development of the standards.

FACT standards define engraftment as the reconstitution of recipient hematopoiesis with blood cells and platelets from a donor. The standards require that policies and procedures be written to describe the review of time to engraftment by the collection facility, processing facility, and clinical transplant program following cellular therapy product administration. Evaluation of engraftment is required to ensure that the highest quality product has been manufactured and distributed. Any unexpected engraftment outcomes should be investigated and corrective aspects or process improvement implemented. Personnel of the clinical transplant program should evaluate all aspects of the collection, processing, and/or administration procedure related to any unexpected engraftment outcome including delayed or failed engraftment. The evaluation should be documented, and corrective action, short and/or long term, be initiated.

Timely engraftment of the hematopoietic progenitor cell (HPC) product in a recipient following a dose-intensive regimen is directly related to the quality of the HPC product. Therefore, the Collection Facility, Processing Facility, and Clinical Transplant Program must be aware of the time to neutrophil and platelet engraftment for all patients for whom they have supplied products. The engraftment information can be solicited directly by the Collection Facility, the Processing Facility, or by another section of the Clinical Transplant Program and presented at a common quality management meeting where select members of the clinical transplant program are in attendance.

There must be evidence of ongoing analysis of engraftment data by the Clinical Transplant Program (see Table 12.1). The analysis should include the average (or median) and observed ranges of engraftment for the various products and transplant procedures performed by the program. The Clinical Transplant Program is the most qualified to determine what constitutes an acceptable time to engraftment and all section of the program should have access to the engraftment data.

Cellular product characteristics, especially CD34 cell dose, should be considered in such analysis. The Collection Facility may consider the number of collections per patient, cell yield per collection, or duration of each collection in its analysis. The Processing Facility may consider white blood cell concentration at the time of cryopreservation, age of the product upon receipt, or viability of the product at time of transplant. These data can be used to identify changes that might require further investigation.

Chimerism assays can be used as a tool for the assessment of the product quality of allogeneic HPC products infused after nonmyeloablative treatment.

TABLE 12.1. Patient/product characteristics considered in engraftment analysis

Collection Facility	Processing Facility	Clinical Transplant Program
Number of collections per patient	CD34+ dose at time of transplant	Number of prior chemotherapy regimens
Cell yield per collection	WBC concentration pre-cryopreservation	Conditioning regimen
Duration of each collection	Age of cellular product	Presence or absence of GVHD
	Viability of cellular product	Disease status
		CMV status

Product efficacy may be more difficult to assess for other nonhematopoietic progenitor cell products, and that assessment will differ for each product type.

Reference

FACT-JACIE International Standards for Cellular Therapy Product Collection, Processing, and Administration (2008).

CHAPTER 13
Follow-Up Care

Carol Jacoby

In caring for the hematopoietic stem cell transplant (HSCT) patient, each transplant center must determine their own programmatic guidelines to ensure the continuity of care of their patients in the immediate post-transplant period. These guidelines typically include anticipated frequency of clinician visits and laboratory assessments, parameters for drug adjustments, and protocols for infectious disease prophylaxis and treatment. Suggestions for follow-up guidelines will be highlighted in this chapter. While institutional standards vary, it is clear that communication with the patient's primary referring oncologist is critical for optimal patient outcomes.

13.1 FOLLOW-UP
1. Clinical evaluations
   a. Autologous transplant patients may be seen in clinic twice weekly until patient is clinically stable, then weekly until day +25−30. Patients may then be seen at 2 week intervals until day +90, monthly for 3 months, every 2 months until 1 year, every 3–6 months for 2–5 years, then annually. At the time of transfer of care to the patient's primary oncologist, recommendations for length of antimicrobial therapy and follow-up should be communicated.
   b. Allogeneic transplant patients may be seen twice weekly through day +50−60, then weekly through day +100. Visits will occur more often for patients with complications. Allogeneic transplant patients after day +100 may be seen at least every 1–2 weeks for 6 months

R.T. Maziarz, S. Slater (eds.), *Blood and Marrow Transplant Handbook*, DOI 10.1007/978-1-4419-7506-5_13, © Springer Science+Business Media, LLC 2011

after transplant, then monthly. Visits should occur more often for patients with chronic graft-versus-host-disease (GvHD) or those individuals with other post-transplant complications. All allogeneic transplant patients should be checked thoroughly for signs and symptoms of GvHD at every follow-up visit.

2. Laboratory studies
   a. Autologous transplant
      i. CBC with differential
      ii. Complete chemistry profile that includes magnesium, renal, LDH, and liver function tests.
      iii. Consider assessment of IgG levels in patients experiencing repeated infections.
      iv. CMV PCR in patients with CD34-selected HSCT procedures
   b. Myeloablative allogeneic transplant
      i. CBC with differential
      ii. Complete chemistry profile that includes renal, liver function studies, LDH, electrolytes, and magnesium.
      iii. CMV by PCR weekly in seropositive recipients, or if donor is seropositive until day +100. (See Chapter 8 for additional CMV monitoring recommendations.)
      iv. Consider surveillance blood cultures weekly while the patient is receiving prednisone ≥ 10 mg/day and has an indwelling catheter. Positive surveillance cultures on asymptomatic patients should be repeated before initiation of antibiotic therapy.
      v. Galactomannan assays weekly through day +100
      vi. IgG levels every other week through day +100. IVIG should be administered per institutional replacement guidelines. If chronic GvHD is present, consider continued monitoring with IVIG replacement per institutional replacement guidelines.
      vii. Calcineurin inhibitor (e.g., cyclosporine or tacrolimus) troughs twice weekly through day +60. Levels can then be followed weekly while receiving therapeutic doses. If the patient is enrolled on a clinical trial, the trough goal may be determined by the protocol. If the patient is not on clinical trial, the trough goal is determined institutionally. An example of a common trough goal is 200–250 ng/dL for cyclosporine and 5–10 ng/dL for tacrolimus. Of note, these blood levels are trough goals (blood drawn approximately 12 h after the last dose).

c. Nonmyeloablative transplant

For patients enrolled on a clinical trial, lab studies should be drawn per study protocol. For patients not receiving care on a clinical trial, consider:

    i. CBC with differential daily until nadir is reached and ANC returns to > 500/mm^3. If the patient's ANC does not go below 500/mm^3, daily CBCs continue until nadir is reached and there is clear increase of ANC × 2 consecutive days. After daily CBCs are no longer needed, check CBC three times weekly until day +28.

    ii. Chemistry profile that includes renal, liver function studies, LDH, electrolytes, and magnesium three times weekly until day +28, then weekly through day +100.

    iii. CMV by PCR weekly until day +100 (see Chapter 8 for additional CMV monitoring recommendations).

    iv. If the patient has GvHD and requires steroid therapy, surveillance blood cultures can be considered weekly as long as the patient is receiving prednisone ≥ 10 mg/day and has an indwelling catheter. Consider repeating cultures prior to initiation of antibiotic therapy on asymptomatic patients.

    v. Galactomannan assays weekly through day +100.

    vi. IgG levels every other week through day +100. IVIG should be administered per institutional replacement guidelines. If chronic GvHD is present, consider continued monitoring with IVIG replacement per institutional replacement guidelines.

    vii. Calcineurin inhibitor trough levels twice weekly until day +56, then discontinued if patient begins a drug taper. Therapeutic calcineurin inhibitor trough levels are typically determined by protocol. A common standard cyclosporine trough goal is 300–400 ng/dL through day +28 and then 250–350 ng/dL from day +28–56; 5–10 ng/dL for tacrolimus. Of note, these blood levels are trough goals (blood drawn approximately 12 h after last dose).

    viii. Consider clinical evaluation and assessment for GvHD at least twice weekly through day +56, then weekly through day +100. Peripheral chimerisms may be drawn on days +28, +56, +84, +180, at 12, 18 months, and then annually for 5 years. Bone marrow biopsy/aspirates can be done on varying schedules. One example includes procedures on days +56 and

+84, then at 6, 12, and 18 months, 2 years, and then annually through year 5. Other follow-up studies are determined by disease state.

13.2 IMMUNOSUPPRESSION

1. Myeloablative transplants
   a. Calcineurin inhibitors and prednisone should be gradually tapered post-transplant. This can be done by decreasing the drugs in a step-wise, linear fashion. As a general rule, immunosuppressive drugs should not be tapered at the same time, but done sequentially.
   b. For patients receiving steroid prophylaxis, consider tapering 10% of the starting steroid dose weekly beginning around day +30–35. A goal would be to have prednisone tapered to 10 mg/daily by day +84.
   c. Calcineurin inhibitors may then be tapered by 10% every week beginning at day +84 as long as there is no active GvHD.
2. Nonmyeloablative transplants
   a. Many trials recommend specific guidelines for tapering of immunosuppressive therapy in the absence of GvHD. An example of a study-driven protocol for immunosuppressive therapy goals on study is as follows:
      i. Sibling-donor transplant patients receive
         – Cellcept (Mycophenolate®) 15 mg/kg po BID through day +28
         – Cyclosporine (Gengraf®, Neoral ®) begins at a dose of 4 mg/kg po BID and is adjusted to maintain a trough goal of 300–400 ng/dL through day +28. The trough goal then decreases to 250–350 ng/dL through day +56. After day +56 if no GvHD is present, patients may begin a 6% per week taper of cyclosporine dose with a goal of ending therapy by day +180.
      ii. Unrelated-donor transplant patients receive
         – Cellcept 15 mg/kg po TID through day +28, then decrease to BID dosing through day +56. Therapy is stopped at day +56.
         – Cyclosporine is started at 4 mg/kg po BID and is adjusted to maintain a trough goal of 300–400 ng/dL through day +28. The trough goal then decreases to 250–350 ng/dl through day +56. After day +56 if no GvHD is present, patients begin a 6% per week taper

of CSA dose with a goal of ending therapy by day +180.

3. Renal insufficiency and Calcineurin inhibitor dosing
   a. Renal function should be followed closely in patients receiving calcineurin inhibitors (see Table 13.1). These drugs are held for serum creatinine levels ≥2.0 mg/dL.
   b. IV hydration may be beneficial to correct an elevated creatinine. Creatinine levels can rise unexpectedly, even in patients who have been receiving calcineurin inhibitor therapy for weeks to months and have had stable renal function.
   c. Calcineurin inhibitors are associated with electrolyte wasting, particularly magnesium. Repletion of magnesium can be accomplished by oral means (dosing may be limited by diarrhea) or by intravenous route.

TABLE 13.1. Dose adjustment for renal insufficiency

Creatinine (mg/dL)	Cyclosporine/tacrolimus taper
1.5–1.75 (or 1–1.5× baseline)	50–75% of current dose
1.76–2 (or 1.6–1.9× baseline)	25–50% of current dose
>2.0 (or >1.9 × baseline)	Hold until creatinine <2.0, then resume at 50–75% of prior dose

13.3 IMMUNIZATIONS

Recommendations for reimmunization are frequently debated and updated. Current opinion suggests treating both autologous and allogeneic patients as though they have never been vaccinated, recommending revaccination for both subsets of patients. Presently, no prevaccination testing is recommended; however, consideration should be given for monitoring immune reconstitution in allogeneic patients prior to vaccination. Reconstitution of the immune system may take months to years and is affected by infection, length of immunosuppressive therapy, and GvHD. The best predictive marker is the peripheral blood CD4+ count; however, following IgG levels will ascertain B-cell function. Alternatively, one could measure antigen-specific antibodies prior to and after administering a killed vaccination to document an appropriate rise in the antibody levels demonstrating a response.

1. General recommendations
   a. The safety of administering live vaccinations is still controversial. However, it is agreed that at a minimum, live vaccines (smallpox, chicken pox [Varivax®, Zostavax®], MMR, yellow fever, and FluMist®) should be avoided for at least 2 years following transplant and for as long as patient is on immunosuppressive therapy. Oral polio vaccine (OPV) is no longer available in the United States, and should be avoided in preference to the injectable polio vaccine (IPV) in stem cell transplant recipients.
   b. Immunization of family members is often recommended and should be based on each transplant center's protocol.
      i. For VZV-seronegative caregivers or those with no history of VZV, it is recommended they receive the VZV vaccination. Isolation from the transplant patient is necessary if the recipient of the vaccine experiences a rash post-vaccination; continue isolation until the rash resolves.
      ii. Family members and close household contacts should receive the trivalent inactivated influenza vaccination every flu season for ~24 months post-HSCT, continuing annually for at least as long as the HSCT recipient remains on immunosuppression.
      iii. HSCT patients should avoid diaper changing of infants and children who receive the Rotavirus vaccine. If this is not possible, practice good hand hygiene.
         – RV5 is dosed at 2, 4, and 6 months of age and is shed in the stool for up to 15 days after vaccination
         – RV1 is dosed at 2 and 4 months of age and is shed in the stool for up to 30 days after vaccination.
      iv. Caregivers and family members over the age of 60 should receive the Zostavax® vaccine. Isolation from the transplant patient is necessary if the recipient of the vaccine experiences a rash post-vaccination; continue isolation until the rash resolves.
      v. Family members may receive MMR vaccine per recommended scheduling. However, they should avoid contact with the HSCT recipient if they develop a fever and/or rash post-vaccination until symptoms resolved.
   c. It is recommended that HSCT recipients receiving immunosuppressive therapy who are exposed to VZV receive VariZig; this is currently only available by an expanded access protocol or compassionate use by the Cangene Corporation in Canada.

i. An alternative option is IVIG if VariZig is not available
2. Immunization-specific recommendations (see Table 13.2)

TABLE 13.2. Vaccination guidelines for adults post-autologous and allogeneic transplant

Months post-transplant	Vaccine	Comments
All live virus vaccines should be avoided if possible. Patients receiving rituximab post-transplant should initiate vaccinations at 12 months post-transplant or 6 months from last rituximab, whichever is later		
3–6	PCV-13	
12	DTaP if available, or Tdap	
	HBV	
	Hib	
	IPV	
	PCV-13	
	Meningococcal conjugate	
14	Td	
	HBV	
	Hib	
	IPV	
18	PCV-13	
24	Td	
	HBV	
	Hib	
	IPV	
	PPSV23	Repeat every 5 years
	MMR	
Annually	Trivalent inactivated influenza vaccine	Begin at 6 months after HSCT; may be given 4 months post-transplant in times of local outbreak. Consider second dose if given <6 months post-transplant

PCV = pneumococcal conjugate vaccine; DTap = full-dose diphtheria, tetanus and acellular pertussis; Tdap = tetanus, reduced-dose diphtheria and reduced-dose pertussis; HBV = hepatitis B; Hib = *Haemophilus influenza*; IPV = inactivated polio; Td = tetanus, diphtheria; PPSV23 = pneumococcal polysaccharide

Table modified from Tomblyn, et al., (2009). Guidelines for preventing infectious complications among hematopoietic cell transplantation recipients; a global perspective. *Biol Blood Marrow Transplant*

a. Pneumococcal vaccine
   i. Timing of initiation of dosing remains controversial.
      – One study showed similar responses in patients vaccinated at 3 months versus 9 months post-transplant.
      – Early vaccination may be preferred as it protects against both early and late pneumococcal infection, but may result in a shorter-lasting antibody response
      – If vaccinations started early, it is crucial to evaluate antibody levels to determine if revaccination is necessary
   ii. PCV-13 is the preferred vaccine for the first 3 doses; however, consider PPSV23 for the fourth dose to provide broader immune response
b. Diphtheria-tetanus vaccine
   i. DT is full-dose diphtheria toxoid while Td is reduced dose. The content of tetanus toxoid is the same in both
   ii. Full toxoid (T) vaccines should be used whenever possible.
   iii. DT vaccine is not currently approved for children >age 7 due to side effects; however, it is usually tolerated well in post-HSCT patients as they are similar to vaccine-naive patients.
   iv. Diphtheria antibody levels after vaccination may be warranted in areas of increased risk of diphtheria.
c. Pertussis vaccine
   i. HSCT patients are more susceptible to complications from pertussis due to underlying pulmonary damage secondary to the conditioning regimen and/or GvHD
   ii. Patients should receive full-dose acellular pertussis toxoid (DTaP); however, in the United States, this vaccine is not approved for patients > 7 years old.
   iii. The Tdap vaccine contains lower doses of diphtheria and pertussis proteins; preliminary data show poor response to Tdap in autologous and allogeneic transplant patients, regardless of timing of the dose.
d. Influenza
   i. Lifelong seasonal vaccination is recommended.
   ii. Begin vaccination at 6 months after HSCT; however, this may be given at 4 months post-transplant in face of local outbreak.
      – The clinician may consider a second vaccination, especially if the first dose was given <6 months post-transplant.

     iii. Use of the trivalent inactivated influenza vaccine is recommended. The live intranasal influenza vaccination (FluMist®) should be avoided.

e. Varicella vaccines
    i. Varivax® (varicella zoster vaccine) should be used when the HSCT patient is at least 2 years post-transplant and is off all immune suppression.
    ii. Zostavax® (herpes zoster vaccine) should be avoided as there is not enough data to assure safety at this time.

f. Hepatitis B vaccine
    i. All HSCT patients should receive hepatitis B vaccines post-transplant
       – For HbsAg- or HbcAg-positive patients, vaccination should be given to prevent the risk of reverse sero-conversion
       – For HbsAg- or HbcAg-negative patients, vaccination should be given to prevent new acquisition of the virus.

g. Meningococcal vaccine
    i. There is a reasonable assumption that conjugated meningococcal vaccines give more stable immune responses than polysaccharide-based vaccines, although no comparative studies have been performed.

h. MMR vaccine
    i. Measles, mumps, and rubella are typically given in a combination vaccine.
    ii. This is a live vaccine; therefore, reimmunization should be considered only when the patient is at least 2 years post-transplant and off all immunosuppressive medications.

i. Human Papillomavirus
    i. Vaccination can be considered in patients who meet age criteria; however, there are no data to support timing of vaccination

13.4 CENTRAL VENOUS CATHETERS

1. In general, autologous transplant patients may have their central catheter removed once their platelet count is consistently >50,000/mm^3 without transfusional support. Assessment of peripheral venous access should be undertaken prior to catheter removal. In patients with very limited peripheral access, the provider should consider retaining their catheters for 90–100 days post-transplant if possible.

2. Allogeneic transplant patients may expect to have a central catheter for at least 3 to 6 months post-transplant, longer if they develop GvHD. It is not uncommon for patients to become bacteremic (symptomatic or asymptomatic) while on immunosuppression therapy. Attempts can be made to sterilize the catheter with appropriate antibiotic therapy. However, in cases of severe sepsis, hemodynamic instability, endocarditis, or persistent bacteremia, the catheter must be removed (see Chapter 14 for additional guidelines).
3. Allogeneic transplant patients with severe cGvHD should maintain venous access.

13.5 ACTIVITIES OF DAILY LIVING GUIDELINES

1. Continue conscientious hand washing.
2. Avoid exposure to contacts with upper respiratory illnesses. If friends/family members are ill, they should not visit. Avoid crowds, but when unavoidable, the HSCT patient should wear a mask. Guidelines vary; however, these recommendations should continue for approximately 30 days post-autologous transplant. For the allogeneic stem cell transplant, a minimum of 60 days is recommended; however, this is also dependent on the patient's dose of immunosuppressive therapy.
3. Avoid all tobacco products and exposure to smoke.
4. Encourage exercise with slow acceleration, as tolerated.
5. No swimming in public or private pools until 2 weeks after central catheter removed and patient is not receiving immunosuppression therapy.
6. Contact with pets (but not feces) is safe with the exception of reptiles, amphibians, and birds. Patients should wash their hands after contact with pets.
7. Gardening (with gloves) is safe after 3 months for autologous patients and 6 months for allogeneic patients without active GvHD.
8. No contact with barnyard animals for at least 6 months after transplant. This timeline should be extended for patients who remain on immunosuppressants. Contact with exotic or wild animals should be avoided for approximately 6 months after autologous transplant and as long as the patient is on immunosuppressive therapy for the allogeneic stem cell transplant patient.
9. Avoid use of pesticides, solvents, or fertilizers for 9–12 months after transplant

10. Return to work or school.
    a. Autologous transplant patients may consider returning to work as early as 3–6 months after transplant. Part-time work is advised for 2–4 months after returning to the work place.
    b. Allogeneic transplant patients may consider returning to work 6–12 months after transplant, if stable. Part-time work is advised for the first 2–6 months after returning to the workplace.
11. Sexual activities
    a. May be resumed after day +30 if the patient has a neutrophil count >1000/mm^3 and a platelet count >50,000/mm^3.
    b. Limiting the number of sexual partners is advised.
    c. Safe sex practices are advised particularly in circumstances of prolonged immune suppression, thrombocytopenia, or epithelial surface/barrier disruption. Condoms should be used for the first year post-transplant.
    d. Vaginal moisturizers, lubricants, or vaginal dilators may be required to preserve vaginal functioning.

13.6 OSTEOPOROSIS

Stem cell patients are at high risk of developing osteoporosis due to multiple predisposing factors.

1. Pre-transplant factors
    a. Age: Men >50, post-menopausal women
    b. Chronic illnesses: anorexia, systemic lupus erythematosis, rheumatoid arthritis, emphysema, end-stage renal disease
    c. Endocrine abnormalities: adrenal insufficiency, Cushing's syndrome, diabetes mellitus, hyperparathyroidism, thyrotoxicosis
    d. GI disorders: celiac disease, GI surgery, inflammatory bowel disease, malabsorption
    e. Hematologic disorders: hemophilia, multiple myeloma, systemic mastocytosis, leukemia, lymphoma, sickle cell disease, thalassemia
    f. Lifestyle factors: smoking, alcohol use (>3 drinks/day), high caffeine intake, inadequate physical activity, vitamin D deficiency, immobility

g. Medications: anticoagulants, anticonvulsants, tacrolimus, cyclosporine, glucocorticoids >5 mg/day or for >3 months, chemotherapy agents (including methotrexate, ifosfamide, cyclophosphamide, doxorubicin, interferon alpha)

2. Post-transplant factors
   a. Immunosuppressive therapy (especially glucocorticoids)
   b. Poor nutrition
   c. Hypogonadism
   d. Inactivity

3. Prevention for allogeneic patients on steroid therapy
   a. At day +60, consider beginning calcium 1,000 mg + vitamin D 1,000 units po TID and bisphosphonate therapy. This therapy should be held if the patient develops GvHD of the GI tract.
      i. Parenteral bisphosphonates
         - Pamidronate (Aredia®) 60–90 mg IV every 3 to 6 months
         - Zolendric acid (Reclast®) 5 mg IV yearly
      ii. Oral bisphosphonates
         - Alendronate (Fosamax®) 70 mg po weekly
         - Ibandronate (Boniva®) 7.5 mg daily or 150 mg monthly
         - Risedronate (Actonel®) 5 mg daily, 35 mg weekly, 75 mg × 2 consecutive days every month, or 150 mg monthly.
      iii. Estrogen/hormone therapy (e.g., Estrace®, Estroderm®, Ortho-EST®, Premarin®, Prempo®). Only indicated for prevention and lowest dose for shortest period of time recommended. Please see prescribing information with specific medication.
      iv. Estrogen agonist/antagonist (Evista®) 60 mg po daily
   b. Consider obtaining a DEXA scan at 1 year post-transplant, then annually if patient remains on glucocorticoid therapy. Discontinue bisphosphonate therapy if DEXA scan is normal and patient is off steroids. DEXA scan should be repeated at age 50 if therapy stopped.
   c. If patient's DEXA scan is consistent with osteoporosis, calcium + vitamin D and bisphosphonates should continue with consideration for the addition of
      i. Parathyroid hormone (teriparatide [Forteo®]) 20 mcg SQ daily. *This medication should not be used in patients with a history of bone metastases,

hypercalcemia, skeletal malignancy, or any history of prior radiation therapy to skeleton.
   ii. Increase vitamin D to 50,000 units po weekly

13.7 SKIN CARE

1. Stem cell transplant patients should use sun block with >15 SPF at all times of sun exposure. Use of sunscreen should be lifelong for all allogeneic transplant patients and those autologous transplant patients who received radiation therapy as part of their conditioning regimen. Skin is more sensitive to sun exposure after radiation or chemotherapy. Skin GvHD can reactivate with sun exposure.
2. Do not go barefoot

13.8 DIET AND FOOD PREPARATION (SEE CHAPTER 7 FOR ADDITIONAL RECOMMENDATIONS)

1. Transplant patients are discouraged from preparing food, particularly early in the transplant course. If they choose to cook for themselves, they should be encouraged to follow all safety recommendations. This includes washing food thoroughly as well as cooking foods to appropriate temperatures. Cooked foods should be refrigerated within 2 h of cooking and then reheated to proper temperatures before eating.
2. A low-bacteria diet is recommended in most stem cell transplant programs to prevent food-borne infections, although there are little clear data to support its benefit. In general, it is felt to be most important when patients are neutropenic or while the patient is on immunosuppressive therapy. The length of time a patient is requested to stay on this diet is varied from 1 to 3 months for autologous and 3 months for allogeneic transplant patients or longer if patients remain on immune-suppressive therapy.

13.9 ENDOCRINE ASSESSMENT

Hypogonadism is prevalent among transplant patients effecting approximately 36% of long-term survivors. It is more common in females than males.

1. Thyroid function tests should be assessed every 6 months post-transplant for all allogeneic transplant patients, and

any patient who received TBI as 30% of patients have been found to be hypothyroid within 18 months of transplant.

2. Testosterone levels or follicle-stimulating hormone (FSH) levels and leutenizing hormone (LH) levels should be drawn at 1 year post-transplant or sooner if patient symptoms require evaluation.

   a. Testosterone replacement may be utilized for patients with low testosterone levels post-transplant if no history or increased risk of prostate cancer

      i. Testosterone is available in several formulations
         - Buccal: 30 mg twice daily
         - Topical: 5–10 gm daily
         - Transdermal: 10–15 mg daily
         - IM: 50–400 mg every 2–4 weeks
         - SL: 5 mg TID

   b. Hormone replacement therapy with cyclic estrogen/progesterone therapy may be helpful for symptoms of early menopause. Sample regimens:

      i. Prempro 1 tablet po daily
      ii. Premarin 0.625–0.25 mg po daily with Provera 2.5–5.0 mg po daily. Women whose uterus remains intact should never receive unopposed estrogen due to increased risk of uterine cancer.
      iii. Yearly/biannual pap smears are recommended along with yearly/biannual mammograms. Women should perform monthly self breast exams and men should perform monthly self testicular exams.

3. For patients with endocrine and/or fertility issues, referral to an endocrinologist, gynecologist, or urologist is appropriate.

13.10 TRAVEL SAFETY

Traveling may expose the autologous transplant patient to many infectious risks; therefore, the patient must be educated to limit his/her exposure. In general, it is safe to start traveling 3–6 months post-transplant, including travel to developing countries. Airline travel is considered safe, but does pose an increased risk of airborne illnesses. Prevention is limited to attempting social distancing from obviously ill passengers and frequent hand washing. Cruise ships are also considered safe; however, the patient must be cognizant of food preparation. It is safest to stay with hot foods, fruits peeled by the patient or family member, processed drinks, hot coffee and/or tea. The patient must be hypervigilant about hand washing throughout the cruise.

Traveling for the allogeneic patient is more restricted if they require chronic immunosuppressive therapy. The same guidelines apply as to the autologous transplant patient; however, it is recommended patients avoid travel to developing countries for a minimum of 1 year post-transplant and, ideally, until all immunosuppressive therapy has been discontinued. Patients should be encouraged to discuss plans for extensive travel with their transplant provider.

For immunization recommendations for the immunocompromised traveler, visit wwwnc.cdc.gov/travel/yellowbook/2010/chapter-8/immunocompromised-traveler.aspx .

References

Abou-Mourad, Y.R., Lau, B.C., Barnett, M.J., Forrest, D.C., Hogge, D.E., Nantel, S.H., et al. (2009). Long term outcome after allo-SCT: Close follow–up on a large cohort treated with myeloablative regimens. *Bone Marrow Transplant*, 45:295–302.

Antin, J.H. (2002). Long-term care after hematopoietic-cell transplantation in adults. *N Engl J Med*, 347:36–42.

Center for Disease Control. Vaccines and Immunizations; Summary of recommendations for Adults, 2010 www.imunize.org/CAT.d/p2011.pdf

Cohen, A., Addesso, V., McMahon, D.J., Staron, R.B., Namerow, P., Maybaum, S., et al. (2006). Discontinuing antiresorptive therapy 1 year after cardiac transplantation: Effect on bone density and bone turnover. *Transplantation*, 81:686–691.

Cohen, A., Shane, E. (2003). Osteoporosis after solid organ and bone marrow transplantation. *Osteoporosis Int*, 14:617–630.

Dykewicz, C.A. (1999). Preventing opportunistic infections in bone marrow transplant recipients. 1(1), 40–49. Published online Jan 2002.

Dykewicz, C.A. (2001). Summary of the guidelines for preventing opportunistic infections among hematopoietic stem cell transplant recipients. *Clin Infect Dis*, 33:143.

Dykewicz, C.A, Jaffe, H.W, Kaplan, J.E. Guidelines for preventing opportunistic infections among hematopoietic stem cell transplant recipients. Recommendations of CDC, the Infectious Disease Society of America, and the American Society of Blood and Marrow Transplantation. www.cdc.gov/mmwr/preview/mmwrhtml/rr4910a1.htm

Lacy, C.F., Armstrong, L.L., Goldman, M.P., Lance, L.L., (Eds.) (2008). *Drug Information Handbook* (17th ed.). Lexi-Comp Inc, Hudson, OH.

National Osteoporosis Foundation. (2010). Clinician guide to prevention and treatment of osteoporosis. National Osteoporosis Foundation, Washington, DC. NOF.org/professionals/pdfs/NOF_clinicianGuide2009_v7.pdf

Pfeilshcifter, J., Diel, I.J. (2000). Osteoporosis due to cancer treatment: Pathogenesis and management. *J Clin Oncol*, 18:1570–1593.

Rizzo, J.D., Wingard, J.R., Tichelli, A., Lee, S.J., Van Lint, M.T., Burns, L.J., et al. (2006). Recommended screening and preventative practices for long-term survivors after hematopoietic cell transplantation; joint recommendation of the European Group for Blood an Marrow Transplantation. Center for International Blood and Marrow Transplant Research, and the American Society for Blood and Marrow Transplantation (EBMT/CIBMTR/ASBMT). *Bone Marrow Transplant*, 37:249–261.

Storek, J., Gooley, T., Witherspoon, R.P., Sullivan, K.M., Storb, R. (1997). Infectious morbidity in long term survivors of allogeneic marrow transplantation is associated with low CD4 T-cell counts. *Am J Hematol*, 131–138.

Syrjala, K.L., Langer, S.L., Abrams, J.R., Storer, B.E., Martin, P.J. (2005). Late effects of hematopoietic cell transplantation among 10 year adult survivors compared with case-matched controls. *J Clin Oncol*, 54:6596–6606.

Tomblyn, M., Chiller, T., Einsele, H., Gress, R., Sepkowitz, K., Storek, J., et al. (2009). Guidelines for preventing infectious complications among HCT recipients. *Biol Blood Marrow Transplant*, 15: 1195–1238.

University of Minnesota Medical Center. The BMT Process. http://www.uofmbmt.org/Adult/TheBMTProcess/c_649319.asp

Yao, S., McCarthy, P.L, Dunford, L.M, Roy, D.M, Brown, K., Pelpham, P., et al. (2008). High prevalence of early-onset osteopenia/osteoporosis after allogeneic stem cell transplantation and improvement after bisphosphonate therapy. *Bone Marrow Transplant*, 41:393–398.

Yokoe, D., Casper, C., Dubberke, E., Lee, G., Munoz, P., Palmore, T., et al. (2009). Safe living after hematopoietic cell transplantation. *Bone Marrow Transplant*, 44:509–519.

PART II
Transplant Complications

CHAPTER 14
Infectious Complications

Lynne Strasfeld

Infections are the most frequently occurring complications of hematopoietic stem cell transplantation (HSCT). Myelosuppressive medications, the conditioning regimen (chemotherapy, radiation therapy), mucosal damage, type of transplant, immune-suppressive therapy, and graft-versus-host disease (GvHD) all predispose the HSCT patient to life-threatening infections. Abnormal B- and T-lymphocyte function results in impaired cellular and humoral immune function. Infections that can occur in the setting of impaired cellular immunity include fungal, protozoal, and viral diseases. Humoral defects can predispose a patient to infection with pyogenic organisms and other bacteria as well as viral infections. Patients are also often hypogammaglobulinemic following transplant. Neutrophil function is impaired by the use of corticosteroids and other medications. Functional asplenia is common. The occurrence of infections in an individual patient varies due to underlying disease and immunosuppression, endogenous host flora, and pretreatment infections. Infections also vary according to the phase of the transplant process.

14.1 TEMPORAL SEQUENCE OF INFECTIONS (SEE FIG. 14.1)

1. First month post-transplant (pre-engraftment, the early period)
   a. *Viral infections* such as herpes simplex virus (HSV), respiratory and enteric viruses, HHV-6 (human herpes virus-6)
   b. *Bacterial infections* caused by both Gram-positive (*Staphylococcus epidermidis*, *Staphylococcus aureus*, and

R.T. Maziarz, S. Slater (eds.), *Blood and Marrow Transplant Handbook*, DOI 10.1007/978-1-4419-7506-5_14, © Springer Science+Business Media, LLC 2011

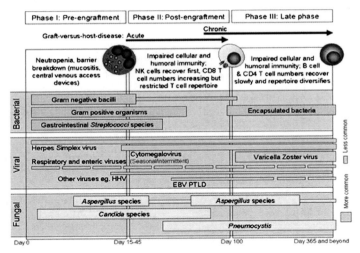

FIG. 14.1. Phases of opportunistic infections among allogeneic HCT recipients. Abbreviations: EBV, Epstein–Barr virus; HHV6, human herpes virus 6; PTLD, post-transplant lymphoproliferative disease. © Granted by Elsevier

> *Streptococcus* species, enterococcus) and Gram-negative organisms (*Klebsiella* species, *Pseudomonas aeruginosa*, and *Escherichia coli*) can result in bacteremia, and perirectal, gastrointestinal tract, skin, and sinopulmonary infections.
>
> c. *Fungal infections*, predominantly *Candida* and *Aspergillus* species

2. 1–4 months post-transplant (post-engraftment, the intermediate period)

   a. *Viral infections*: CMV, respiratory and enteric viruses, BK virus, and HHV-6 can cause infection of the sinopulmonary, central nervous system, gastrointestinal, hepatic, and urogenital systems, depending on the causative organism.

   b. *Bacterial infections*: Gram-positive and Gram-negative organisms. Primarily, these infections arise from the skin, sinopulmonary system, or the gastrointestinal tract.

   c. *Fungal infections* can be caused by a number of organisms such as *Candida*, *Aspergillus*, *Zygomycetes*, *Cryptococcus* species, and reactivation of endemic fungi (e.g., coccidioidomycosis). These infections typically involve the sinopulmonary, central nervous system, liver, spleen, mouth, and/or integumentary system. *Pneumocystis jiroveci* pneumonia can occur in particular in patients on suboptimal *Pneumocystis* prophylaxis.

d. *Protozoal infections*: *Toxoplasma gondii* can affect the central nervous system most commonly, or present in a disseminated fashion.

3. 4–12 months post-transplant (late period)
   a. *Viral infections* may continue to cause serious infections with the most common viral illness being varicella zoster virus (VZV), community-acquired respiratory and enteric infections, and CMV infection in patients with GvHD and prior history of early post-transplant CMV reactivation/infection.
   b. *Bacterial infections* caused by encapsulated organisms (e.g., *Streptococcus pneumonia*, *Haemophilus influenzae*)
   c. *Fungal infections*, both yeasts and molds, may occur, particularly in those patients who remain on immunosuppressive therapy, have GVHD and/or CMV infection. *Pneumocystis* pneumonia can occur in particular in patients on suboptimal *Pneumocystis* prophylaxis.
   d. *Protozoal infections*: *Toxoplasma gondii* can affect the central nervous system most commonly or present in a disseminated fashion.

4. Greater than 12 months post-transplant
   a. *Viral infections* are primarily integumentary VZV infections, community-acquired respiratory and enteric infections, and CMV infection in patients with chronic GvHD and prior history of CMV reactivation/infection.
   b. *Bacterial infections* are primarily induced by encapsulated organisms.
   c. *Fungal infections*, both yeasts and molds, may be a problem, particularly in those patients who remain on immunosuppressive therapy, have GvHD, and/or CMV infection.
   d. *Protozoal infections* can occur late as well, again primarily in patients who remain on immunosuppressive therapy.

14.2 EMPIRIC ANTIMICROBIAL THERAPY AND EVALUATION OF NEUTROPENIC FEVER

1. Neutropenic fever protocol
   a. For the first neutropenic fever ($T \geq 38°C$)
      i. Blood cultures from all lumens of central catheter as well as peripheral draw

ii. UA dip/micro and urine culture

iii. Sputum culture if patient is coughing and able to expectorate sample

iv. 2-view CXR to evaluate for pulmonary infection

v. Discontinue prophylactic oral antibiotics (e.g., fluoroquinolone)

vi. Begin empiric parenteral antibiotic therapy with coverage for Gram-negative organisms as soon as possible, and always within 1 h of the initial fever

– Autologous recipients should receive an anti-Pseudomonal third- or fourth-generation cephalosporin (e.g., cefepime* 2 g IV q 8 h) or, in particular if the patient has been on third/fourth-generation cephalosporin as prophylaxis, a carbapenem (e.g., meropenem 1 g IV q 8 or imipenem 500 mg IV q 6)*

– Nonmyeloablative allogeneic recipients should receive an anti-Pseudomonal third- or fourth-generation cephalosporin (e.g., cefepime* 2 g IV q 8 h) or, in particular if the patient has been on third/fourth-generation cephalosporin as prophylaxis, a carbapenem (e.g., meropenem 1 g IV q 8 or imipenem 500 mg IV q 6)*

– Ablative allogeneic recipients should receive a carbapenem (e.g., meropenem 1 g IV q 8 or imipenem 500 mg IV q 6)*

– Antibiotics should be given through alternating ports of central venous catheter

– For septic/clinically unstable patients, consider broadening empiric regimen to include an aminoglycoside (e.g., tobramycin* 5 mg/kg dosing preferred) as well as extended Gram-positive coverage (see point 2 in Section 14.2)

* Note: Consideration of the local institutional antibiogram as well as any patient-specific history of prior drug-resistant bacteria is critically important in determining the empiric antibiotic selection.

b. For subsequent fevers

i. For $T \geq 38°C$, draw one set of cultures every 24 h. If the patient has a triple lumen catheter, select a different port with each culture set that is drawn.

ii. After three consecutive blood cultures have been drawn at least 24 h apart, cultures should be drawn with any clinical deterioration and at the discretion of the provider.

iii. Draw blood cultures prior to any empiric antibiotic change.

iv. If the patient has been afebrile for at least 48 h and develops a new fever $\geq 38^\circ$C, draw one set of blood cultures.

c. Adjustment of empiric antibiotic regimen

i. If cultures are positive, ensure regimen is appropriate based on pathogen susceptibility pattern.

ii. Discontinue empiric antibiotic therapy once ANC $\geq$ 500 cells/mm^3 if patient remains afebrile and there is no documented infection. A "last on, first off" approach to withdrawal of empiric antibiotics is reasonable, though in practice there is a great deal of variability regarding order and timing of antibiotic discontinuation.

2. Indications for use of empiric extended Gram-positive coverage for neutropenic fever

a. Add vancomycin for any patient with:

i. sepsis (and NOT previously known to be colonized/infected with vancomycin-resistant *enterococcus* [VRE])

ii. documented infection with a Gram-positive organism while awaiting identification and results of susceptibility testing (GPC clusters on culture or GPC pairs/chains for patient NOT previously known to be VRE colonized/infected)

iii. suspicion for skin or central venous catheter source (cellulitis, phlebitis)

iv. history of methicillin-resistant *Staphylococcus aureus* (MRSA) colonization/infection

v. febrile patient with grade II–IV mucositis

b. For patients known to be VRE colonized/infected, use daptomycin* as extended Gram-positive agent in the setting of sepsis and/or Gram-positive bacteremia (GPC in pairs and/or chains) while awaiting pathogen identification and susceptibility pattern. Given the potential for myelosuppression with use of linezolid, daptomycin is the preferred agent in this setting.

* Note: Daptomycin should NOT be used for treatment of pneumonia (in setting of pneumonia and need for VRE coverage, consider use of linezolid).

   c. Blood and wound cultures (when applicable) should be obtained prior to adding vancomycin or daptomycin (or linezolid).

   d. Discontinue vancomycin or daptomycin (or linezolid) after 72 h if no Gram-positive organisms have been cultured and patient has no evidence of shock, pneumonia, or skin/central venous catheter source, regardless of presence or absence of fever.

3. Management of persistent neutropenic fevers (>72 h after initiation of empiric antibacterial therapy)

   a. For patients who are receiving fluconazole, change therapy to voriconazole 6 mg/kg IV × 2 doses, then 4 mg/kg IV/po q 12 h.

     i. Alternatives should voriconazole be contraindicated (e.g., liver enzyme abnormalities, drug–drug interactions) include:
- lipid-based amphotericin 3–5 mg/kg IV q 24
- echinocandin:
  - micafungin 100 mg IV daily
  - caspofungin 70 mg IV load × 1 dose, then 50 mg IV daily
  - anidulafungin 200 mg IV load × 1 dose, then 100 mg IV daily

   b. For patients who are receiving posaconazole prophylaxis, check a noncontrast CT chest, serum galactomannan, and consider sending a posaconazole level.

     i. If the CT chest is suspicious for fungal infection or the serum galactomannan is positive, switch to voriconazole with dosing as above and consult Pulmonary Service for consideration of diagnostic bronchoscopy.

     ii. Patients with symptoms of sinusitis should also have CT sinus screen and ENT evaluation when indicated.

   c. If a patient is receiving voriconazole and has suspicion for invasive mold infection, consider malabsorption of voriconazole (check voriconazole level prior to drug discontinuation) or a voriconazole-resistant organism, and consider change to lipid-based amphotericin product (Ambisome® or Abelcet®).

     i. Indications for the use of Ambisome® in lieu of Abelcet® (based on financial considerations, presuming this is a more costly alternative) include:
- concomitant use of other nephrotoxic agents
- central nervous system fungal infection

    ii. Patients who do not meet the above criteria can receive Abelcet®

d. Clinical evaluation should determine whether an echinocandin (as dosed above in point 3.a in Section 14.2) should be added (e.g., septic picture, suspicion of Candidemia with azole-resistant *Candida* species). If added, this drug should be discontinued and azole prophylaxis/empiric therapy resumed if an alternative explanation for fevers is identified.

4. Criteria for removal of central venous catheters

  a. Central venous catheters should be removed for positive blood cultures with the following organisms

    i. *Staphylococcus aureus*

    ii. *Pseudomonas aeruginosa*

    iii. *Candida* species

    iv. *Fusarium* species

    v. any multi-drug-resistant Gram-negative organism

    vi. mycobacterial species

  b. Clinical criteria necessitating removal of central venous catheters includes

    i. septic patient with line source suspected

    ii. tunnel infection

    iii. failure of response (persistent bacteremia, with positive blood cultures after 48 h of appropriate antibiotic therapy)

14.3 TREATMENT OF COMMON SPECIFIC INFECTIONS IN THE STEM CELL PATIENT POPULATION

Of paramount importance in the treatment of infections in the HSCT recipient is the ability to obtain an accurate diagnosis. Symptoms of infection may be nonspecific or even attenuated in the heavily immunosuppressed HSCT recipient. Diagnosis of infection may require culture of blood or other body fluid, molecular diagnostics (e.g., PCR), radiographic study, invasive diagnostics to obtain tissue or other material (for culture, molecular diagnostics, biomarker study, and pathologic examination), as well as careful ongoing assessment for change in clinical status.

1. Herpes zoster infection

  a. May be localized to a single dermatome or disseminated (see Fig. 14.2). A thorough skin examination is recommended to evaluate for disseminated disease.

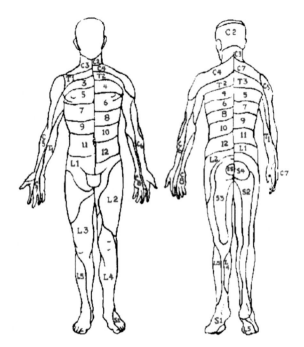

FIG. 14.2. Dermatome map for determination of the extent of herpes zoster infections

    b. Typically occurs 4–5 months post-transplant (or later in allogeneic transplant patients) and may be associated with visceral or central nervous system disease.

    c. Treatment with high-dose acyclovir (10 mg/kg IV every 8 h) until lesions are completely crusted is warranted in patients with visceral or disseminated disease or who are on immunosuppressive therapy.

    d. Oral antiviral therapy with acyclovir 800 mg po 5 times daily is the standard of care for lesions confined to a single dermatome. Valacyclovir (Valtrex®) 1,000 mg po TID may be used as an alternative to oral acyclovir and is likely to achieve better therapeutic plasma levels against VZV. Although this agent is not licensed for use in HSCT recipients in the United States, there are reasonable safety data on its use in this patient population.

e. While active against VZV, limited safety and efficacy data on use of famciclovir (Famvir®) in the HSCT population preclude recommendation for use in this setting.

f. For severe herpes zoster infections (>1 dermatome, trigeminal nerve involvement or disseminated disease), patients require hospitalization and should receive intravenous acyclovir (10 mg/kg IV every 8 h) until lesions have completely crusted and no new lesions are evident, then conversion to an oral compound (acyclovir or valacyclovir) to complete the treatment course. Dosing should be adjusted for renal function. Monitor renal function and encephalopathy as adverse effects of high-dose acyclovir.

g. If the patient is allergic to acyclovir or resistance is suspected, therapy should be changed to foscarnet 40 mg/kg IV every 8 h until lesions are completely crusted and no new lesions are evident. Dosing needs to be adjusted for renal function.

2. Herpes simplex virus (HSV) infection

a. Caused by HSV type 1 or 2, with type 1 more often affecting skin and mucous membranes (including eyes) above umbilicus and type 2 more often affecting skin and mucous membranes below the umbilicus.

b. For a first episode, oral antiviral therapy is usually adequate with acyclovir 400 mg po 5 times daily for 14–21 days. If the patient is unable to tolerate oral medications, change to acyclovir 5 mg/kg IV every 8 h for 7 days.

c. For recurrent episodes, patient should receive acyclovir 400 mg po TID for 5–10 days. Alternative therapy includes valacyclovir 500 mg po BID for 5–10 days.

d. While active against HSV, limited safety and efficacy data on use of famciclovir in the HSCT population preclude recommendation for use in this setting.

e. Some patients may require chronic suppression due to frequently recurring outbreaks. Any of the following medications is acceptable therapy: acyclovir 400–800 mg po BID–TID or valacyclovir 500 mg po BID.

f. Dosing for suspected/proven HSV encephalitis is acyclovir 10 mg/kg IV every 8 h, adjusted for renal function, for a total of 21 days.

3. Human herpes virus-type 6 (HHV-6) infection

a. Reactivation can lead to encephalitis in the post-transplant period.

  b. PCR testing (CSF, blood) should be performed; MRI of the brain may reveal abnormalities, often times involving the medial temporal lobes.

  c. Treatment is controversial, but for established encephalitis, foscarnet or ganciclovir should be used in therapeutic doses. Treatment decisions should be made on a case-by-case basis in consultation with the Infectious Diseases Consultation Service.

4. Cytomegalovirus (CMV) infection

  a. CMV infection can lead to end-organ disease in the HSCT recipient, manifesting as pneumonia, gastroenteritis, hepatitis, myelosuppression, retinitis, and/or encephalitis.

  b. Diagnosis may require diagnostic bronchoscopy and/or tissue biopsy. Blood for quantitative PCR and fluid/tissue for CMV culture may help in establishing the diagnosis. Consider that CMV PCR detection in blood may not be fully sensitive for detection of end-organ disease, in particular with gastrointestinal disease. Tissue biopsy should be obtained when possible if CMV disease is suspected.

  c. If CMV end-organ disease is suspected/proven, recommend consultation with the Infectious Diseases Consultation Service for patient-specific treatment recommendations. First-line therapy for CMV disease is generally with IV ganciclovir, with foscarnet reserved for cases with intolerance to ganciclovir (refractory cytopenias) or if ganciclovir-resistance is suspected (i.e., if CMV viral load increases while on therapy for more than 2 weeks) or documented. Ganciclovir-resistant virus is an unusual occurrence in the HSCT population and most often occurs in patients who have had prolonged exposure to ganciclovir or valganciclovir. Dosing duration should be determined on a case-by-case basis, based on the extent of CMV disease and the immune status of the host. Generally, induction dosing (see Chapter 8) should be given for at least 3 weeks, until the CMV viral load is at or near undetectable and until symptoms of end-organ disease have resolved, with several weeks of maintenance IV ganciclovir or oral valganciclovir dosing thereafter. For CMV pneumonia, in addition to antiviral therapy, adjuvant IVIG 500 mg/kg IV every other day for 10 doses should be given.

5. Adenovirus and BK virus infections of the genitourinary tract
    a. Both adenovirus and BK virus can result in hemorrhagic cystitis post-transplant.
    b. For patients who develop BK viral cystitis, supportive care measures should be instituted initially. Begin with antispasmotics such as oxybutinin or urinary tract analgesics such as phenazopyridine. Consider reducing immune suppression if able and begin continuous bladder irrigation if symptoms are not controlled with antispasmotics. For patients who develop fulminant hemorrhagic cystitis, consider therapy with cidofovir 1 mg/kg IV weekly to 3 times weekly without probenecid. Firm data on dosing and efficacy are not available at this time. Viral load quantification does not correlate with symptoms, and the clinical significance of the viral load is unknown. Important adverse drug effects associated with cidofovir administration include nephrotoxicity as well as hematologic and ocular toxicity; therefore, careful monitoring is recommended in this setting.
    c. Adenovirus is also a potential cause of hemorrhagic cystitis, but is significantly more likely than BK virus to result in disseminated disease and is therefore associated with a greater risk of mortality. Adenovirus can affect the lungs, gastrointestinal tract, liver, genitourinary system, and/or the central nervous system. Patients who have a positive culture or PCR for adenovirus from their urine should have blood sent for quantitative adenovirus . If this is positive and/or if patient has fulminant hemorrhagic cystitis, strong consideration should be given to treatment with cidofovir 5 mg/kg IV once weekly for 2 weeks, then every other week or 1 mg/kg IV three times weekly. If systemic or disseminated disease is suspected, add probenecid 2 g orally 3 h prior to cidofovir dose, then 1 g orally at 2 and 8 h after dose.
6. Respiratory viral infections
    a. The most common respiratory viruses seen in the post-HSCT patient population are parainfluenza (serotypes 1–4, especially serotype 3) respiratory syncytial virus (RSV), influenza, adenovirus, rhinovirus, and human metapneumovirus.
    b. Testing for respiratory viral infections should be by molecular methods/multiplex PCR from nasopharyngeal

sample or lower respiratory tract sample, as this offers the highest sensitivity for diagnosis. Evaluation of suspected lower respiratory tract infection in patients with upper respiratory tract infection (URI) should include CT scan of the chest.

c. Droplet and contact precautions should be initiated with either suspicion for or documented respiratory viral infection. These precautions should continue until the patient is asymptomatic and repeat testing for viral infection is negative. If inhalational ribavirin is used, patient must be in a negative airflow room with respiratory isolation.

d. Parainfluenza
   i. If nasal washings/nasopharyngeal swab is positive for parainfluenza, obtain a chest CT if lower respiratory tract infection (LRTI) is suspected.
   ii. If lower tract disease is evident, consider treating with IVIG 500 mg/kg IV every other day, though noting the data supporting this measure are very limited.

e. RSV
   i. All patients who have nasal washings positive for RSV should have a CT scan of the chest without contrast to evaluate for lower tract disease.
   ii. If the CT chest is negative, the absolute lymphocyte count (ALC) is > 300 cells/mm^3 and the steroid dose is <0.5 mg/kg/day (prednisone equivalent), no treatment is required.
   iii. If the CT chest is consistent with LRTI, patients should receive ribavirin 20 mg/mL (2 g over 6 h every 8 h) × 7 days using a Viratek small particle generator (SPAG-2) by face mask or endotracheal tube, regardless of their absolute lymphocyte count or steroid dose. IVIG 500 mg/kg QOD × 5 doses should be given to any patient with LRTI.
   iv. Consider inhalational ribavirin therapy along with IVIG administration, as above, for any allogeneic recipient with RSV URI with an ALC < 300 cells/mm^3 or steroid dose >0.5 mg/kg/day (prednisone equivalent), with the goal of preventing progression to LRTI.

f. Influenza A and B
   i. Initiate therapy with an appropriate antiviral agent, as empiric antiviral therapy for influenza will vary

depending on the drug-resistance patterns of circulating strains. Consultation with Infectious Diseases is strongly recommended.

ii. Influenza vaccination with the inactivated vaccine is recommended for all HSCT recipients (autologous patients ≥100 days post-transplant and allogeneic patients ≥180 days post-transplant) and for caregivers of HSCT recipients. Efficacy of vaccination post-transplant is highly dependent on host immune status, a function of the time since transplant and the immune suppressive regimen.

iii. Unvaccinated caregivers and patients who have been exposed to influenza should be referred for chemoprophylaxis as soon as possible, and within 48 h of the exposure. Drug-resistance patterns of the circulating influenza strain should guide the choice of antiviral prophylaxis.

iv. In the context of a significant community outbreak or transmission on the transplant unit/in the transplant clinic, policies for chemoprophylaxis should be discussed with the Infectious Diseases Consultation Service/Infection Control and considered based on drug-resistance patterns of the circulating influenza strain.

g. Adenovirus

i. Cidofovir should be strongly considered in the context of invasive adenovirus infection. While data on optimal dosing of cidofovir are not available, the usual practice is to use 5 mg/kg IV once weekly for 2 weeks and then every other week in the setting of life-threatening or disseminated disease, along with probenecid 2 g orally 3 h prior to cidofovir dose, then 1 g orally at 2 and 8 h after dose. Important adverse drug effects associated with cidofovir administration include nephrotoxicity as well as hematologic and ocular toxicity, and so careful monitoring is recommended in this setting.

ii. When possible, immunosuppression should be reduced in the setting of life-threatening or disseminated adenovirus disease.

iii. The use of adjuvant intravenous immunoglobulin can be considered in the treatment of life-threatening or disseminated infection, though the data supporting this approach are limited.

7. Epstein-Barr virus (EBV)
   a. Fever, adenopathy, and extranodal disease may occur. Quantitative EBV PCR from blood, tissue, and immunohistochemistry on tissue samples are helpful in diagnosis.
   b. EBV-DNA load monitoring has been recommended by some for certain high-risk HSCT recipients, although the threshold for preemptive intervention is not clear. Patients who received T-cell depleted or haplo-identical marrows, or who have been exposed to ATG should have quantitative EBV PCR monitoring every 2 weeks.
   c. First-line therapy for established PTLD is the administration of anti-CD20 monoclonal antibody, rituximab. Infusion of EBV-specific cytotoxic T-lymphocytes has been used with success, though this requires significant time for in vitro generation. There is little evidence to support the contribution of antiviral therapy for this indication.
8. Viral hepatitis
   a. Patients who are hepatitis B virus (HBV) surface antigen and/or HBV DNA positive should be evaluated by hepatology and/or the Infectious Diseases Consultation Service, with consideration for liver biopsy prior to transplant as well as antiviral therapy prior to proceeding with the transplant conditioning regimen. During the course of antiviral therapy, HBV DNA should be monitored to ensure suppression, in particular in the setting of abnormal liver function tests. Antiviral therapy should be continued for at least 6 months post-transplant in autologous recipients and at least 6 months following discontinuation of immunosuppressive therapy in allogeneic recipients.
   b. Patients who are hepatitis C virus (HCV) prior to transplant should be evaluated by hepatology for evidence of underlying cirrhosis, with a liver biopsy when indicated. Those patients with documented cirrhosis or hepatic fibrosis should receive a conditioning regimen that does not contain either cyclophosphamide or total body irradiation, as those regimens pose an increased risk of hepatic sinusoidal obstruction syndrome. Treatment for chronic HCV should be considered in HSCT recipients who are in remission from their underlying disease, ≥2 years post-transplant without active GvHD, and off immunosuppression for 6 months.

9. *Pneumocystis jiroveci* pneumonia (PCP)

a. Infection is rare in patients compliant with first-line PCP prophylaxis (such as trimethoprim-sulfamethoxazole) but breakthrough infections are possible, in particular in patients on other than first-line agents. Radiographic studies of the chest (CT and CXR) typically reveal a diffuse interstitial infiltrate with ground glass appearance, although appearance can be quite varied.

b. First-line treatment is trimethoprim-sulfamethoxazole 15–20 mg/kg/day (need to renal dose adjust with abnormal renal function) of IV trimethoprim equivalent divided into 3–4 daily doses for 21 days.

c. If patient is sulfa-allergic, alternative therapies include pentamidine 4 mg/kg/day IV (need to renal dose adjust with abnormal renal function) for 21 days (for severe disease) or clindamycin 450 mg po q 6 h with primaquine 15 mg (base) po daily (for mild to moderate disease) for 21 days. Corticosteroids at a dose of 40 mg po BID days 1–5, then 40 mg po daily for days 6–10 and 20 mg po daily for days 11–21 can be considered in combination with antimicrobial therapy if patient not already receiving steroids in comparable dosages in the setting of moderate to severe disease.

d. Unique side effects associated with daily pentamidine therapy include hypotension, hypo/hyperglycemia, pancreatitis, and/or cardiac arrhythmias.

10. *Toxoplasma gondii* Infection

a. Fifteen to thirty percent of US population has been previously infected, as evidenced by positive serostatus. The risk of toxoplasmosis following allogeneic HSCT depends on the seroprevalence in the population and on the conditioning regimen, with a report of toxoplasmosis reactivation in 8.7% of donor and/or recipient-seropositive myeloablative transplantations. This organism most often affects the central nervous system, but can also be a cause of disseminated infection in HSCT recipients. A CT or MRI of the brain may reveal focal mass lesion(s) or, less commonly, diffuse encephalitis. If toxoplasmosis is suspected, check PCR (CSF and/or blood) and serology. Tissue samples should be obtained when possible to aid in diagnosis.

b. Treatment of established disease due to toxoplasmosis is with pyrimethamine 200 mg po on day 1, then 75 mg po daily and sulfadiazine 6 gm/day po divided q 6 h, with folinic acid 10 mg po daily.

c. Alternatives include trimethoprim-sulfamethoxazole 10 mg/kg/day po divided q 12 h or pyrimethamine with folinic acid + either clindamycin 600 mg po q6, clarithromycin 1 g po bid or azithromycin 1.2–1.5 g q po 24, or atovaquone 750 mg po q 6.

d. Treatment should continue for 4–6 weeks following resolution of signs and symptoms of active infection, then thereafter a course of suppressive therapy.

11. Infections with *Candida* species

a. Infections can be classified as primarily superficial (cutaneous or mucosal) or invasive (e.g., candidemia, hepatosplenic candidiasis).

b. Oropharyngeal candidiasis

Treatment is primarily aimed at local application with the use of nystatin 5–10 mL (100,000 units/mL) swish and spit/swallow QID, clotrimazole troches 10 mg dissolved in mouth 4–5 times per day, or amphotericin rinse (50 mg/200 mL sterile water) 5–10 mL swish and spit QID. More complicated infections may require azole or echinocandin therapy.

c. Esophageal candidiasis

Fluconazole 200–400 mg/day po/IV for 14–21 days is first line in azole-inexperienced individuals. In patients with significant antecedent azole exposure or for fluconazole-refractory disease, an extended spectrum azole (e.g., posaconazole 400 mg po BID or voriconazole 200 mg po BID) or an echinocandin (e.g., micafungin 150 mg daily) can be used.

d. Vulvovaginal candidiasis

Fluconazole 100–200 mg/day po/IV for 7–10 days or topical antifungal treatment (e.g., clotrimazole, miconazole, or nystatin) for 7–10 days will usually clear the infection.

e. Candida cystitis

i. Consider whether this is a contaminant or an infection, based on whether the patient is displaying signs and/or symptoms of UTI. If the patient has an indwelling catheter, change out the catheter and repeat urine studies.

ii. Treatment of candiduria is indicated, regardless of presence/absence of symptoms, in neutropenic hosts.

iii. Fluconazole 200 mg po/IV daily for 7–14 days is the treatment of choice for candida cystitis for fluconazole-sensitive organisms.

iv. For treatment of cystitis due to fluconazole-resistant organisms (e.g., *C. krusei* and *C. glabrata*), amphotericin-based products (either systemic administration or by bladder irrigation) can be used. Voriconazole is not an effective drug for candidal cystitis, given that active drug is not excreted to the urine in significant amount.

v. Although the echinocandins achieve low concentrations in the urine, there is limited data describing successful use of these antifungal agents for treatment of renal parenchymal infections.

vi. In patients with recurrent or seemingly complicated *Candida* cystitis, a renal ultrasound should be performed to evaluate for the possible presence of a fungal mass, which would entail surgical debridement along with systemic antifungal therapy for cure.

f. Candidemia

i. An echinocandin (e.g., micafungin 100 mg IV daily) or an amphotericin B lipid-based product (dose 3–5 mg/kg IV daily) is recommended for neutropenic hosts with candidemia, while awaiting species-level identification, which can guide further therapy. For patients who are not critically ill and without recent azole exposure, high-dose fluconazole 800 mg po/IV loading dose, followed by 400 mg po/IV daily or voriconazole 6 mg/kg po BID for 2 doses as load, followed by 3 mg/kg po BID can be considered.

ii. For infections due to *C. albicans* or *C. parapsilosis*, either fluconazole or an amphotericin-based product is acceptable, with fluconazole a less toxic and more convenient choice once the patient has stabilized.

iii. For infections due to *C. glabrata*, an echinocandin is preferred, with amphotericin-based therapy a less attractive option in light of the potential for toxicity.

iv. For infections due *to C. krusei*, either an echinocandin, voriconazole, or a lipid formulation of amphotericin is acceptable.

v. Removal of vascular catheter is advised in this setting.

vi. An ophthalmology consultation should be obtained to evaluate for *Candida* endophthalmitis. A CT of the abdomen should be considered to evaluate for hepatosplenic candidiasis (see below) in the appropriate setting. With high-grade and persistent candidemia, an echocardiogram should be obtained to evaluate for endocarditis.

g. Chronic disseminated candidiasis

i. This syndrome, also referred to as hepatosplenic candidiasis, is most often seen during recovery from neutropenia.

ii. Diagnosis is suggested by an elevation of the serum alkaline phosphatase and/or multiple hepatic hypodensities seen on imaging of the abdominal viscera. Blood cultures are typically negative.

iii. Treatment considerations include azole therapy (most often fluconazole, as *C. albicans* is the species most commonly implicated in this setting), an echinocandin, or a lipid-based amphoteracin product. The bulk of available data is with amphotericin B deoxycolate and fluconazole. Treatment decision should be based on previous antifungal therapy and microbiologic data when available.

12. Invasive aspergillosis

a. Pulmonary infection is the most common presentation, but disease can also affect the central nervous system, sinuses, skin, and at times result in other organ involvement in the setting of hematogenous dissemination. *Aspergillus fumigatus* is the most common species implicated as a cause of infection in HSCT recipients and other immunocompromised hosts, although other species can also result in invasive infection.

b. Key to successful management is early consideration of this process, with imaging and appropriate diagnostic maneuvers, along with prompt initiation of antifungal therapy.

c. Diagnosis can often be established with use of *Aspergillus* galactomannan testing on bronchoalveolar lavage fluid. When a diagnosis cannot be obtained by less invasive means, surgical biopsy should be considered.

d. Voriconazole 6 mg/kg IV q 12 h × 2 doses, then 4 mg/kg IV/po q 12 h is the first-line therapy for invasive aspergillosis. Voriconazole trough levels should be measured early (3–7 days after initiation of therapy) in any patient with proven or probable invasive aspergillosis, or with a poor response to treatment, possible side effects of therapy, suspicion of poor oral absorption, or complex drug–drug interactions. Target trough level range is ~2 to 5–6 mcg/mL.

e. If a significant increase in transaminase levels is noted while on voriconazole therapy (≥ 5 times the upper limit of normal), send a voriconazole trough value and change therapy to a lipid-based amphotericin product or posaconazole (with close monitoring of liver enzymes).

f. A phase 4 clinical trial of combination therapy (voriconazole along with an echinocandin) in this setting is ongoing to determine whether combination therapy is superior to voriconazole monotherapy. At the present time, the routine use of combination therapy to treat pulmonary aspergillosis is not recommended.

g. Reduction of immunosuppression is advised (especially taper or withdrawal of corticosteroids), when possible, in patients with invasive aspergillosis.

h. Surgical resection should be considered when pulmonary lesions are in close proximity to the great vessels or pericardium, with persistent hemoptysis from a single cavitary lesion, with pericardial infection or chest wall invasion.

i. The use of recombinant human growth factors such as filgrastim or sargramostim may be helpful in this population, primarily in the neutropenic patient. A prospective study to determine the utility of granulocyte transfusions in this setting is ongoing.

j. Patients with a history of invasive aspergillosis prior to transplant should receive at least 6 weeks of antifungal therapy and have a documented partial or complete response to therapy before conditioning. Ideally, these patients should be steered toward a non-myeloablative regimen. Secondary prophylaxis with an anti-*Aspergillus* azole (voricoanzole or posaconazole) should be given to patients in the post-allogeneic HSCT setting. If significant drug–drug interactions or drug toxicity limit azole use, lipid-based amphotericin products or echinocandins can be used as a second-line approach in this setting.

13. Other fungal Infections

a. While non-aspergillosis mold infections are relatively uncommon, there are other molds to consider in this patient population.

    i. Zygomycosis is increasingly recognized in highly immunosuppressed HSCT recipients. Iron chelation with deferoxamine predisposes to infection. Clinical presentation may include angioinvasive infection of the lungs, skin, brain, and widespread visceral involvement in the setting of disseminated disease. Management of this infection should entail antifungal therapy, reversal of underlying defects in host defense (tapering of immunosuppression and restoration of euglycemia) when possible, and surgical debridement where applicable. Lipid formulations of amphotericin B 5–10 mg/kg/day IV are first-line antifungal therapy. Posaconazole 200 mg po QID or 400 mg po BID is a second-line option for salvage therapy or for secondary prophylaxis. Voriconazole does not have activity against mucormycosis. Despite aggressive management of this infection, mortality rates remain very high. Consultation with the Infectious Diseases Service is suggested.

    ii. Disseminated fusariosis in highly immunosuppressed HSCT recipients is often characterized by cutaneous lesions and positive blood cultures, with or without visceral involvement. Antifungal susceptibility is varies by species. Treatment of disseminated infection is with either voriconazole (if organism is other than *Fusarium solani* or *F. verticillioides*) or with an amphotericin B product. In addition to antifungal treatment, management should include surgical debridement when applicable as well as improvement in host immune response. Prognosis is generally poor and is determined to a large extent by the degree of immunosuppression. Growth factor support and/or granulocyte transfusions can be considered as adjuvants to care in persistently neutropenic individuals. Consultation with the Infectious Diseases Service is suggested.

  b. Cryptococcosis is reported uncommonly in the HSCT population. This may well relate to widespread use of azole prophylaxis in this patient population. Cryptococcal infection may result in pulmonary, central nervous system, cutaneous, or widely disseminated infection. Diagnostic work-up should include lumbar puncture when this entity is considered. Management is with lipid formulations of amphotericin B or fluconazole, along with serial lumbar puncture in the context of cryptococcal meningitis. Concurrent use of flucytosine is often avoided in HSCT recipients, given the potential for marrow toxicity. Consultation with the Infectious Diseases Service is suggested.

c. While relatively uncommon, the endemic mycoses (coccidioidomycosis, histoplasmosis, and blastomycosis) should be considered as either reactivation or new infection in patients from endemic areas. Evaluation may include serologic tests as well as culture and biopsy. Antifungal treatment is variable and dependent on the extent of infection. Consultation with the Infectious Diseases Service is suggested.

References

Boeckh, M. (2008). The challenge of respiratory virus infections in hematopoietic cell transplant recipients. *Br J Haematol*, 143: 455–467.

Cesaro, S., Hirsch, H.H., Faraci, M., et al. (2009). Cidofovir for BK virus-associated hemorrhagic cystitis: A retrospective study. *Clin Infect Dis*, 49:233–240.

Emanuel, D., Cunningham, I., Jules-Elysee, K., et al. (1988). Cytomegalovirus pneumonia after bone marrow transplantation successfully treated with the combination of ganciclovir and high-dose intravenous immune globulin. *Ann Intern Med*, 109:777–782.

Foo, H., Gottlieb, T. (2007). Lack of cross-hepatotoxicity between voriconazole and posaconazole. *Clin Infect Dis*, 45:803–805.

Fricker-Hidalgo, H., Bulabois, C.E., Brenier-Pinchart, M.P., et al. (2009). Diagnosis of toxoplasmosis after allogeneic stem cell transplantation: Results of DNA detection and serological techniques. *Clin Infect Dis*, 48:e9–e15.

Hughes, W.T., Armstrong, D., Bodey, G.P., et al. (2002) 2002 guidelines for the use of antimicrobial agents in neutropenic patients with cancer. *Clin Infect Dis*, 34:730–751.

Ison, M.G. (2006). Adenovirus infections in transplant recipients. *Clin Infect Dis*, 43:331–339.

Jones, J.L., Kruszon-Moran, D., Wilson, M., McQuillan, G., Navin, T., McAuley, J.B. (2001). Toxoplasma gondii infection in the United States: seroprevalence and risk factors. *Am J Epidemiol*, 154: 357–365.

Kontoyiannis, D.P., Marr, K.A., Park, B.J., et al. (2010). Prospective surveillance for invasive fungal infections in hematopoietic stem cell transplant recipients, 2001–2006: Overview of the Transplant-Associated Infection Surveillance Network (TRANSNET) Database. *Clin Infect Dis*, 50:1091–1100.

Lee, W.M., Grindle, K., Pappas, T., et al. (2007). High-throughput, sensitive, and accurate multiplex PCR microsphere flow cytometry system for large-scale comprehensive detection of respiratory viruses. *J Clin Microbiol*, 45:2626–2634.

Ljungman, P., de la Camara, R., Cordonnier, C., et al. (2008). Management of CMV, HHV-6, HHV-7 and Kaposi-sarcoma herpes virus (HHV-8) infections in patients with hematological malignancies and after SCT. *Bone Marrow Transplant*, 42: 227–240.

Ljungman, P., de la Camara, R., Milpied, N., et al. (2002). Randomized study of valacyclovir as prophylaxis against cytomegalovirus reactivation in recipients of allogeneic bone marrow transplants. *Blood*, 99:3050–3056.

Martino, R., Parody, R., Fukuda, T., et al. (2006). Impact of the intensity of the pretransplantation conditioning regimen in patients with prior invasive aspergillosis undergoing allogeneic hematopoietic stem cell transplantation: A retrospective survey of the Infectious Diseases Working Party of the European Group for Blood and Marrow Transplantation. *Blood*, 108:2928–2936.

McDonald, G.B. (2006). Review article: management of hepatic disease following haematopoietic cell transplant. *Aliment Pharmacol Ther*, 24:441–452.

Meers, S., Lagrou, K., Theunissen, K., et al. (2010). Myeloablative conditioning predisposes patients for Toxoplasma gondii reactivation after allogeneic stem cell transplantation. *Clin Infect Dis*, 50:1127–1134.

Mermel, L.A., Allon, M., Bouza, E., et al. (2009). Clinical practice guidelines for the diagnosis and management of intravascular catheter-related infection: 2009 Update by the Infectious Diseases Society of America. *Clin Infect Dis*, 49:1–45.

Musher, B., Fredricks, D., Leisenring, W., Balajee, S.A., Smith, C., Marr, K.A. (2004). Aspergillus galactomannan enzyme immunoassay and quantitative PCR for diagnosis of invasive aspergillosis with bronchoalveolar lavage fluid. *J Clin Microbiol*, 42:5517–5522.

Nucci, M., Anaissie, E. (2007). Fusarium infections in immunocompromised patients. *Clin Microbiol Rev*, 20:695–704.

Pappas, P.G., Kauffman, C.A., Andes, D., et al. (2009). Clinical practice guidelines for the management of candidiasis: 2009 update by the Infectious Diseases Society of America, *Clin Infect Dis*, 48:503–535.

Pascual, A., Calandra, T., Bolay, S., Buclin, T., Bille, J., Marchetti, O. (2008). Voriconazole therapeutic drug monitoring in patients with invasive mycoses improves efficacy and safety outcomes. *Clin Infect Dis*, 46:201–211.

Perfect, J.R., Cox, G.M., Lee, J.Y., et al. (2001). The impact of culture isolation of Aspergillus species: A hospital-based survey of aspergillosis. *Clin Infect Dis*, 33:1824–1833.

Reed, E.C., Bowden, R.A., Dandliker, P.S., Lilleby, K.E., Meyers, J.D. (1988). Treatment of cytomegalovirus pneumonia with ganciclovir and intravenous cytomegalovirus immunoglobulin in patients with bone marrow transplants. *Ann Intern Med*, 109:783–788.

Savona, M.R., Newton, D., Frame, D., Levine, J.E., Mineishi, S., Kaul, D.R. (2007). Low-dose cidofovir treatment of BK virus-associated hemorrhagic cystitis in recipients of hematopoietic stem cell transplant. *Bone Marrow Transplant*, 39:783–787.

Schmidt, G.M,. Kovacs, A., Zaia, J.A., et al. (1988). Ganciclovir/immunoglobulin combination therapy for the treatment of human cytomegalovirus-associated interstitial pneumonia in bone marrow allograft recipients. *Transplantation*, 46:905–907.

Smith, J., Andes, D. (2008). Therapeutic drug monitoring of antifungals: pharmacokinetic and pharmacodynamic considerations. *Ther Drug Monit*, 30:167–172.

Sobel, J.D., Bradshaw, S.K., Lipka, C.J., Kartsonis, N.A. (2007). Caspofungin in the treatment of symptomatic candiduria. *Clin Infect Dis*, 44:e46–49.

Spellberg, B., Walsh, T.J., Kontoyiannis, D.P., Edwards, J. Jr., Ibrahim, A.S. (2009). Recent advances in the management of mucormycosis: from bench to bedside. *Clin Infect Dis*, 48:1743–1751.

Styczynski, J., Einsele, H., Gil, L., Ljungman, P. (2009). Outcome of treatment of Epstein-Barr virus related post-transplant lymphoproliferative disorder in hematopoietic stem cell recipients: A comprehensive review of reported cases. *Transpl Infect Dis*, 11:383–392.

Sun, H.Y., Wagener, M.M., Singh, N. (2009). Cryptococcosis in solid-organ, hematopoietic stem cell, and tissue transplant recipients: evidence-based evolving trends. *Clin Infect Dis*, 48:1566–1576.

Tomblyn, M., Chiller, T., Einsele, H., et al. (2009). Guidelines for preventing infectious complications among hematopoietic cell transplantation recipients: a global perspective. *Biol Blood Marrow Transplant*, 15:1143–1238.

Walsh, T.J., Anaissie, E.J., Denning, D.W., et al. (2008). Treatment of aspergillosis: clinical practice guidelines of the Infectious Diseases Society of America. *Clin Infect Dis*, 46:327–360.

Weinstock, D.M., Ambrossi, G.G., Brennan, C., Kiehn, T.E., Jakubowski, A. (2006). Preemptive diagnosis and treatment of Epstein-Barr virus-associated post transplant lymphoproliferative disorder after hematopoietic stem cell transplant: an approach in development. *Bone Marrow Transplant*, 37:539–546.

CHAPTER 15
Acute Graft-Versus-Host Disease

Susan Slater

Despite advances in HLA typing, acute GvHD remains a leading cause of morbidity and mortality among allogeneic transplant recipients. It is estimated that 30–50% of patients who receive stem cell products from HLA-identical siblings will develop grades 2–4 GvHD, while rates of GvHD in matched unrelated donor transplants are estimated to be between 50 and 70%. Acute GvHD has historically been defined as occurring prior to day +100 and chronic GvHD as occurring after day +100. However, recently there has been a move to define GvHD based on the clinical symptoms and pathologic findings rather than by an arbitrary timeline. The outcome of acute GvHD is dependent on the overall grade of GvHD and the patient's response to initial treatment.

15.1 PATHOPHYSIOLOGY
Three conditions are felt to contribute to the development of acute GvHD:

1. The patient must receive an infusion of immune-competent donor cells.
2. There must be an immunologic disparity between the recipient and the donor cells.
3. The recipient must be unable to mount an appropriate immune response to these "foreign" cells, at least long enough for the donor cells to engraft and mount an anti-host immunologic response.

The development of GvHD is described as a three-part process:

R.T. Maziarz, S. Slater (eds.), *Blood and Marrow Transplant Handbook*, DOI 10.1007/978-1-4419-7506-5_15, © Springer Science+Business Media, LLC 2011

1. Tissue damage occurs as a consequence of the patient's malignancy, prior therapies, and/or the transplant conditioning regimen. This injury results in the release of inflammatory cytokines such as TNF-α, IL-1, and IL-2, leading to activation of the recipient's antigen-presenting cells (APCs).
2. These inflammatory cytokines and both patient and donor APCs interact with donor T-cells, leading to T-cell expansion and release of additional inflammatory cytokines.
3. These activated T-cells produce inflammatory cytokines and cellular mediators, resulting in apoptosis in the target host cells, typically within the skin, gut, and liver target tissues.

15.2 RISK FACTORS

1. Recipient age
2. Stem cell source (marrow > PBSC > cord blood)
3. HLA disparity of donor and recipient
4. $CD34^+$ cell dose $>6 \times 10^6$
5. Immune-suppressive regimen for GvHD prophylaxis (CSA > tacrolimus)
6. Diagnosis of CML (possibly related to better functioning APCs due to minimal prior therapy)
7. CMV negative status

Note: Historically risk factors for GvHD have also included allosensitized donors (heavily transfused, prior pregnancy) and sex mismatched donor/recipient; however, more recent studies have found these etiologic factors not statistically significant.

15.3 INCIDENCE

1. The median time to onset for symptoms of acute GvHD is approximately 3 weeks, with a range of 1–14 weeks.
2. An estimated 30–50% of sibling-donor recipients and 50–70% of unrelated-donor recipients will develop grades 2–4 GvHD.
   a. Skin is usually the first organ involved and often coincides with engraftment.
   b. Of patients who develop GvHD, approximately 80% will have skin involvement, 50% gut involvement, and 50% liver involvement.
3. For patients alive at 60 days post-transplant, only 5–8% will subsequently develop acute GvHD.

15.4 CLINICAL PRESENTATION

Onset of symptoms typically occurs 2–3 weeks after transplant. The primary organs affected by acute GvHD are the skin, liver, and GI tract.

1. *Skin*: Classically manifests as an erythematous, maculopapular rash ± pruritus involving the pinnae, palms, and soles. This rash often spreads to involve the neck and trunk, with later involvement of the extremities. Severity is determined by percentage of BSA involved (see Fig. 15.1) and may range from a mild, non-pruritic rash to bullous formation and desquamation reminiscent of toxic epidermal necrolysis.

2. *Liver*: An elevated serum bilirubin is the typical manifestation of liver involvement, although elevated alkaline phosphatase may also be an indicator of impending disease. A variant of liver GvHD has also been described, which manifests as hepatitis with transaminitis and elevated alkaline phosphatase; however, these are not classic findings and are not specific.

3. *GI*: Manifestations include anorexia, nausea, vomiting, diarrhea, and/or abdominal cramping; however, these are

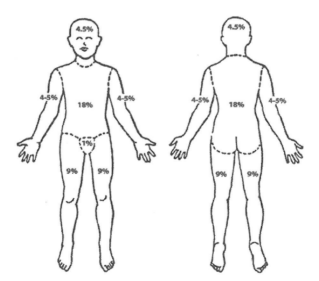

FIG. 15.1. Rule of nines (Body Surface Area)

relatively nonspecific findings and may be attributed to the conditioning regimen, immune-suppressive medications, or infections.

15.5 EVALUATION AND DIAGNOSIS

Tissue pathology is the gold standard for diagnosis of GvHD. Clinical correlation is necessary as many non-GvHD causes (damage from conditioning regimen, infection, drug eruptions, viral exanthems) may mimic the pathologic findings of GvHD (see Table 15.1).

1. Skin:
   a. Dermatology consult for skin biopsy. Criteria for diagnosis of GvHD include evidence of basal vacuolization, necrotic epidermal cells, lymphocytes in the dermis, and exocytosis in the epidermis.
2. Liver:
   a. Liver ultrasound to r/o SOS, cholelithiasis
   b. Consider liver biopsy for tissue diagnosis, either ultrasound guided percutaneous or transjugular, if patient is thrombocytopenic.
3. GI:
   a. Stools to r/o *Clostridium difficile* and other enteral pathogens
   b. GI consult for endoscopy. There is no clear correlation between endoscopic findings and GvHD stage.
   c. To make the diagnosis of GvHD, apoptosis must be present on pathology review; however, this finding is not exclusive to GvHD.

15.6 STAGING/GRADING

Standardized staging of GvHD is critical to evaluating extent of disease, response to therapy and prognosis. The most widely used Glucksberg staging criteria, developed in 1974, is organ-specific and based on percentage of body surface area (BSA) involved, volume of diarrhea, and/or total bilirubin (Table 15.2). These stages are then evaluated together, in combination with performance status, to determine an overall grade of GvHD (Table 15.3).

There have been attempts to modify the Glucksberg system to identify a correlation of patterns of organ involvement with

TABLE 15.1. Findings associated with acute GvHD

Organ	Clinical manifestations	Histologic findings	Alternate diagnoses
Skin	Erythematous maculopapular rash involving the palms, soles, pinnae, spreading to the trunk and later extremities. ± pruritus. Bullae/desquamation in severe cases	Basal vacuolization, necrotic epidermal cells, lymphocytes in dermis, exocytosis in epithelium	Chemotherapy/radiation effect Drug eruption Viral exanthem Infection
Liver	Hyperbilirubinemia, jaundice. Possible hepatitis with transaminitis, elevated alkaline phosphatase	Bile duct damage, bile duct lymphocytic infiltration, endothelialitis	Sinusoidal obstructive syndrome Medication effect Extrahepatic obstruction TPN Infection Iron overload
GI	Anorexia, nausea, vomiting, diarrhea, abdominal pain/ileus, GI bleeding	Apoptosis, crypt cell necrosis and drop out, epithelial denudation	Chemotherapy/radiation effect GI tract infection (C. difficile, CMV, etc.) Drug reaction

treatment-related mortality and treatment failure. In 1997, the CIBMTR developed a Severity Index (Table 15.4), which graded GvHD based on organ involvement alone and grouping patients with similar risks of treatment-related morbidity and treatment failure. While the original Glucksberg criteria remain the most commonly used staging system, the CIBMTR staging criteria is increasingly being adopted. For patients receiving therapy on study protocols, one should become familiar with the staging system associated with that protocol to ensure accurate and consistent measurements of GvHD.

TABLE 15.2. Glucksberg organ staging

Stage	Skin	Liver (bilirubin)	Gut (stool output/day)
0	No rash	<2 mg/dL	<500 mL/day or persistent nausea
1	Maculopapular rash =25% BSA	2–3 mg/dL	>500 mL/day
2	Maculopapular rash 25–50% BSA	3.1–6 mg/dL	>1000 mL/day
3	Generalized erythroderma	6–15 mg/dL	>1500 mL/day
4	Generalized erythroderma + bullous formation	>15 mg/dL	Severe abdominal pain, ± ileus, ± bleeding

TABLE 15.3. Glucksberg overall grading

Grade	Skin	Liver	Gut	ECOG performance
I	Stage 1–2	Stage 0	Stage 0	0
II	Stage 1–3	Stage 1 and/or	Stage 1	0–1
III	Stage 2–3	Stage 2–3 and/or	Stage 2–3	2–3
VI	Stage 2–4	Stage 2–4 and/or	Stage 2–4	3–4

TABLE 15.4. CIBMTR severity index

	Skin		Liver		GI	
Index	Stage (Max)	Extent of rash	Stage (Max)	Bilirubin (μmol/L)	Stage (Max)	Diarrhea (mL/day)
A	1	<25%	0	<34	0	<500
B	2	25–50% or	1–2	34–102 or	1–2	500–1500
C	3	>50% or	3	103–255 or	3	>1500
D	4	Bullae or	4	>255 or	4	Pain, ileus

Patients who develop grade 1 or 2 acute GvHD have an 80% probability of long-term survival. Survivorship falls to 30% for patients with grade 3 disease and 5% for patients with grade 4 disease.

15.7 TREATMENT (SEE CHAPTER 9 FOR DISCUSSION OF GVHD PROPHYLAXIS)

1. General guidelines
   a. The standard mainstay of treatment for acute GvHD is corticosteroids; however, there is no consensus on initial dosing or tapering schedule.
      i. Should patient's rash progress to >50% of BSA or patient develop GvHD involving the gut or liver, systemic steroids should be dosed at 1–2 mg/kg/day depending on the current stage and potential predicted severity of GvHD.
      ii. For patients with stage 1 and 2 disease, there is no evidence that beginning with 1 mg/kg/day of steroid has led to worse patient outcomes overall. Additionally, no benefit has been shown with steroid doses >2 mg/kg/day.
   b. Maximize benefit of calcineurin inhibitors in combination with steroids by maintaining therapeutic drug levels (CSA ~200 ng/mL, tacrolimus ~8–10 ng/mL)
   c. To avoid potential side effects of protracted high-dose steroids, tapering should begin after 7 days of therapy regardless of response. There are no clear guidelines for steroid tapering. One could consider a stepwise decrease by 0.25 mg/kg/day every 5–7 days to a dose of 1 mg/kg/day, then continue to decrease by 10% every 7 days as tolerated.
   d. The most important predictor of long-term survival is response to high-dose steroids. Complete responses are seen in approximately 25–40% of patients with steroids alone, while 40–50% of patients will achieve a partial response. Due to infection and organ failure, steroid refractory disease is associated with a high rate of morbidity and mortality.
   e. Ensure adequate antifungal and antiviral prophylactics are in place (see Chapter 8 for prophylaxis guidelines). Change to IV formulation if absorption is questionable due to diarrhea.
      i. Acyclovir 800 mg po BID or 250 mg/m^2 IV daily
         – Weekly monitoring of CMV PCRs remains critical as GvHD often precipitates CMV reactivation (see Chapter 8 for monitoring guidelines and treatment recommendations)
      ii. Maximize fungal coverage:

- Posaconazole (Noxifil®) 200 mg po TID; however, this medication is contraindicated in patients with GI GvHD due to absorption issues.
- Voriconazole (VFend®) 4 mg/kg po/IV BID
- If patient is unable to tolerate azoles due to transaminitis, consider low-dose liposomal amphotericin 1 mg/kg IV daily or 3 mg/kg IV three times weekly

2. Organ specific
   a. Skin
      i. Stage 1 and 2 skin GvHD can be treated with topical steroids such as triamcinolone 0.1% or betamethasone 0.1% cream or ointment. These moderate-dose topical steroids should be used only on the trunk and extremities. Hydrocortisone 1% is safe for application to the face, neck, and groin. If possible, wrap affected areas after application to provide occlusion to increase absorption.
      ii. Emollients to prevent breakdown of dry and fissured skin areas
      iii. Keep skin clean and dry, using gentle hypoallergenic soaps
      iv. Antipruritic agents (diphenhydramine 12.5–50 mg po q 6 h, hydroxyzine 25 mg po QID)
   b. Liver
      i. Hold medications which may contribute to hyperbilirubinemia (particularly azoles)
      ii. Consider ursodiol 300 mg po BID to increase water solubility of bile salts and protect liver cells from toxic bile acids
   c. GI
      i. NPO or stage I GvHD diet depending on symptoms
      ii. IV hydration. Consider TPN early depending on severity of symptoms
      iii. Change all immune suppression to IV formulation to ensure absorption
      iv. Supportive care for antiemetics and antidiarrheals
      v. Consider Gram-negative prophylaxis or anaerobic protection in light of compromised mucosal integrity
         - Ciprofloxacin 500 mg po BID or 400 mg IV BID
         - Imipenem 500 mg IV q 6 h

15.8 STEROID REFRACTORY DISEASE

There is no standard definition of steroid refractory GvHD; however, failure of therapy has been defined as progression of symptoms after 3 days of high-dose steroids or no improvement after 7 days of therapy. Approximately 40% of sibling-donor and 25% of unrelated-donor transplant patients will respond to therapy; 60–75% of patients will require additional therapy. There is also no consensus on the best salvage therapy for steroid refractory disease. Multiple agents have been utilized with varying degrees of success (see Table 15.5).

1. Antithymocyte globulin (ATG)
   a. ATGAM® (equine)
      i. *Mechanism of action*: Affects cell mediated immunity by selectively destroying lymphocytes
      ii. *Dosing and administration*:
         – Despite the fact that historically, ATG is the most commonly used second-line therapy, no standard regimen has been identified. ATG preparations should not be used interchangeably as their potency differs. Dosing examples: 10–15 mg/kg IV QOD × 6–7 doses; 15 mg IV BID × 8–10 doses; 30 mg/kg IV QOD × 6 doses; 15 mg/kg IV daily × 12 doses; or 40 mg/kg IV daily × 4 days.
         – A test dose is recommended prior to the first dose of ATG. Inject 0.1 mL of a 1:1,000 dilution intradermally into one arm with a control of 0.1 mL NS into the contralateral arm. A systemic reaction including rash, tachycardia, dyspnea, hypotention, or anaphylaxis is a contraindication for administration of the drug. If a wheal and/or erythema >10 mm occurs, consider an alternative therapy.
         – Pre-medicate for all doses (excluding test dose) with acetaminophen 650 mg po, diphenhydramine 50 mg IV, and methylprednisolone (or equivalent) 50–100 mg IV.
         – Meperidine 12.5–25 mg IV q 1 h prn rigors.
      iii. *Adverse effects*:
         – Sepsis
         – Anaphylaxis
         – Serum sickness
         – Dyspnea, pulmonary edema
         – Chest/back pain

TABLE 15.5. Agents for salvage therapy in steroid refractory GvHD

Drug	Class	Dose/route	Preferred use	FDA approval
Alemtuxumab (Campath®)	MAB	10 mg IV/day × 5 doses	Skin, liver	B-cell chronic lymphocytic leukemia
ATG – equine (ATGAM®)	Immune serum	No defined standard dosing	Skin, GI, liver	Aplastic anemia; prevention/treatment of renal transplant rejection
ATG – rabbit (Thymoglobulin®)	Immune suppressant	2.5 mg/kg IV × 4–6 days or 2.5 mg/kg QOD on days 1, 3, 5, and 7	Skin, GI, liver	Renal transplant rejection
Basiliximab	MAB	No defined standard dosing	Skin	Prevention/treatment of renal transplant rejection
Beclomethasone (orBec®)	Adrenal glucocorticoid	2 mg po q 6 h of both immediate release and enteric-coated capsules	GI only	Crohn's Disease
Budesonide (Entocort®)	Adrenal glucocorticoid	3 mg po TID or 9 mg po daily	GI only	
Denileukin diftitox (Ontak®)	IL-2	9 mcg/kg IV on days 1, 3, 5, 15, 17, and 19	Skin, liver	Primary cutaneous T-cell lymphoma, CD25+
Etanercept (Enbrel®)	TNF inhibitor	25 mg SQ twice weekly × 4–8 weeks	GI	Ankylosing spondylitis, chronic plaque psoriasis, RA, juvenile idiopathic arthritis

TABLE 15.5. (*Continued*)

Drug	Class	Dose/route	Preferred use	FDA approval
Extracorporeal photopheresis	n/a	n/a	Skin. liver	
Infliximab	TNF inhibitor	10 mg/kg/day IV weekly × 1–4 weeks	GI	Ankylosing spondylitis, chronic plaque psoriasis, RA, Crohn's, ulcerative colitis
Inolimomab	MAB	11 mg/day × 3 days or 5.5 mg/day IV for 7 days, then 5.5 mg IV QOD × 5 doses	Skin, liver	Investigational
Mycophenolate mofetil (Cellcept®)	Immune suppressant	1.5–3 g po daily in two divided doses	Skin, liver	Prevention/treatment of rejection in cardiac, renal & liver transplant
Pentostatin (Nipent®)	Antimetabolite, antineoplastic	1.5 mg/m^2 on days 1–3 and 15–17	Skin, GI, liver	Hairy cell leukemia
Sirolimus (Rapamune®)	Bacterial macrolide antibiotic	15 mg/m^2 po load on day 1, then 5 mg/m^2 po daily × 13 days or 4–5 mg/m^2 po daily × 14 days without a loading dose; adjust dose to maintain a trough level of 4–12 ng/mL.	Skin, GI, liver	Prevention/treatment of rejection in renal transplant

MAB = monoclonal antibody; IL-2 = interleukin 2; TNF = tumor necrosis factor

- Leukopenia, thrombocytopenia
- Rash, urticatia
- Fever, rigors
- N/V/D
- Renal function abnormalities
- Extravasation may result in tissue necrosis and nerve damage

b. Thymoglobulin® (rabbit)

  i. *Mechanism of action*: Affects cell-mediated immunity by selectively destroying lymphocytes

  ii. *Dose and administration*:
   - No standardized dosing has been established: 2.5 mg/kg IV daily × 4–6 days; 2.5 mg/kg IV on days 1, 3, 5, and 7 are included within the various schedules that have been reported.
   - No test dose is required
   - Pre-medicate for all doses with acetaminophen 650 mg po, diphenhydramine 50 mg IV, and methylprednisolone (or equivalent) 50–100 mg IV.
   - Meperidine 12.5–25 mg IV q 1 h prn rigors.

  iii. *Adverse effects*:
   - CMV reactivation, sepsis
   - Abdominal pain, N/V/D
   - Hypertension, tachyarrhythmias
   - Fever, rigors
   - Leukopenia, thrombocytopenia
   - Myalgias
   - Dyspnea
   - Dizziness, headaches

2. Denileukin diftitox (Ontak®)

  a. *Mechanism of action*: A fusion protein that introduces diphtheria toxin into cells that express IL2 receptor (antiCD25), inhibiting cellular protein synthesis which results in T-cell death.

  b. *Dose and administration*: 9 mcg/kg IV, over 1 h, on days 1, 3, 5, 15, 17, and 19, is a dose schedule commonly used. Pre-medicate 60 min prior to infusion with acetaminophen 650 mg po, diphenhydramine 25–50 mg po/IV and dexamethasone 8 mg IV.

  c. *Adverse effects*: BLACK BOX WARNING: Serious and fatal infusion reactions may occur; maintain emergency medications at bedside including diphenhydramine 25–50 mg IV q 2 h prn, dexamethasone 4 mg IV × 1 prn and epinephrine 1:1000, 0.3 mg SQ q 20 min prn. Capillary leak syndrome resulting in death may also occur (but has been observed more frequently when the medication is given in higher doses).

    i. Pulmonary edema
    ii. Rash/pruritus
    iii. Anorexia, N/V/D
    iv. Transaminitis
    v. Arthralgias/myalgias
    vi. Headaches, weakness
    vii. Dyspnea, cough
    viii. Reduced visual acuity
    ix. Constitutional symptoms of fever/rigors, fatigue

3. Etanercept (Enbrel®)
    a. *Mechanism of action*: Dimeric soluble TNF receptor that inactivates TNF-α and TNF-β.
    b. *Dose and administration*: 25 mg SQ twice weekly for 4–8 weeks
    c. *Adverse effects*: BLACK BOX WARNING: Increased risk for serious infections, including bacterial sepsis, invasive fungal, and other opportunistic infections.
        i. Abdominal pain, N/V
        ii. Headache
        iii. Injection site reaction
        iv. Rhinitis/URI
        v. Rare complications include cytopenias, aplastic anemia, Stevens-Johnson syndrome, autoimmune hepatitis, malignant lymphoma (children > adults)

4. Extracorporeal photopheresis (ECP)
    a. *Mechanism of action*: No definitive mechanism of action has been identified. The leading hypothesis involves induction of cellular apoptosis, which results in modulation of antigen-presenting cell activation inducing immune tolerance and increased production of regulatory T-cells.
    b. *Procedure*:
        i. Through leukopheresis, a patient's blood is removed and then centrifuged. 8-methoxypsoralen is added to the buffy coat/plasma, which is then exposed to a UVA light source prior to being returned to the patient.
        ii. ECP is administered in multiple schedules. One typical schedule is that ECP is performed on two consecutive days, every 1–4 weeks for varying lengths of time depending on patient's response.

   c. *Adverse effects*:
     i. Vasovagal syncope/hypotension
     ii. Anemia/thrombocytopenia
     iii. Bleeding secondary to procedure-related anticoagulant
     iv. Central venous catheter-associated bacterial infections/sepsis Constitutional symptoms of nausea, fever/chills, headache
5. Monoclonal antibodies
   a. Alemtuzumab (Campath$^{®}$)
     i. *Mechanism of action*: Binds to cell surface CD52, which is present on all B- and T-lymphocytes, resulting in cell lysis.
     ii. *Dose and administration*: 10 mg/day IV × 5 doses
     iii. *Adverse effects*:
        – Increased risk of infection, specifically CMV reactivation/infection, EBV, and sepsis
        – EBV-associated lymphoproliferative disorder, tumor lysis syndrome, or progressive multifocal leukoencephalopathy
        – Autoimmune hemolytic anemia/thrombocytopenia
        – Cardiomyopathy, CHF, cardiac dysrhythmia
        – Pancytopenia
        – Guillain–Barre syndrome
        – Toxic optic neuropathy
        – Goodpasture's syndrome (rapidly progressive glomerulonephritis with pulmonary hemorrhage)
        – Rash, urticaria
        – N/V/D
        – Bronchospasm, dyspnea
   b. Infliximab (Remicade$^{®}$)
     i. *Mechanism of action*: Binds to soluble and transmembrane forms of TNF-α, neutralizing its activity and causing cell lysis.
     ii. *Dose and administration*: 10 mg/kg/day IV weekly for 1–4 weeks
     iii. *Adverse effects*: BLACK BOX WARNING: Increased risk for serious infections, including bacterial sepsis, invasive fungal, and other opportunistic infections. Rare cases of hepatosplenic T-cell lymphoma, usually fatal, have been reported in patients with Crohn's disease and ulcerative colitis treated with infliximab and who were concurrently receiving treatment with azathioprine or 6-mercaptopurine

- Acute coronary syndrome
- Erythema multiforme, Stevens–Johnson syndrome
- Pancytopenia
- Demyelinating disease of the CNS
- Abdominal pain, nausea
- Headache
- Fatigue
- Rare complications include hepatotoxicity, drug-induced lupus erythematosis, immune hypersensitivity reaction.

c. Inolimomab

i. *Mechanism of action*: A murine anti-IL-2 receptor, which blocks activation of the alpha-chain of the IL-2 receptor (CD25); this may inhibit IL-2-mediated T-cell activation.

ii. *Dose and administration*: 11 mg/day IV × 3 days, 5.5 mg/day IV × 7 days, then 5.5 mg IV QOD × 5 doses per manufacturer's instructions. The optimum dose and duration of therapy have yet to be determined.

iii. *Adverse effects*:

- Human antimouse antibody responses occur frequently (allergic reaction to the mouse antibodies ranging from a mild rash to ARF). There is no clear evidence of decreased effectiveness of the drug.
- Rates of infection are comparable to standard immune suppression alone.

d. Basiliximab (Simulect®)

i. *Mechanism of action*: An IL-2 receptor antagonist that inhibits IL-2 binding, preventing IL-2mediated activation of lymphocytes and impairing immune response.

ii. *Dose and administration*: No standardized dose has yet been defined. In trials, various doses have been used with varied response. Additional studies are necessary to determine appropriate dosing.

iii. *Adverse effects*:

- Acute allergic reaction
- CMV reactivation/infection
- Candidiasis
- Dysuria
- Cough, dyspnea
- Edema
- Hypertension
- Abdominal pain, vomiting
- Dizziness, weakness

   e. Daclizumab (Zenepax®)

      i. Per Hoffmann-La Roche, Inc. production of daclizumab has been discontinued in the United States due to decreased demand and available alternative treatments. The lots of daclizumab for the United States market will expire in 2011.

6. Mycophenolate mofetil (Cellcept®, MMF)

   a. *Mechanism of action*: The active metabolite, mycophenolic acid, inhibits the synthesis pathway of guanosine nucleotides, resulting in selective suppression of B- and T-cell proliferation and possibly preventing the recruitment of leukocytes to sites of inflammation.

   b. *Dose and administration*: 1.5–3 g po or IV daily in two divided doses. IV and po dosing are equivalent.

   c. *Adverse effects*:

      i. Hypertension, peripheral edema

      ii. Hyperlipidemia

      iii. Electrolyte abnormalities

      iv. Increased risk of opportunistic infection

      v. Abdominal pain, N/V/D/C

      vi. Weakness, headache, insomnia

      vii. Increased frequency of UTIs, renal function abnormalities

      viii. Dyspnea, cough, pleural effusions, pulmonary fibrosis

      ix. Pancytopenia

      x. Progressive multifocal leukoencephalopathy

      xi. Rare complications include gastric ulceration/perforation

7. Nonabsorbable corticosteroids

   a. Beclomethasone (orBec®)

      i. *Mechanism of action*: A synthetic corticosteroid with potent glucocorticoid, but weak mineralocorticoid activity. The mechanism of its anti-inflammatory effects has not been clearly established.

      ii. *Dose and administration*: 2 mg po q 6 h of both immediate release and enteric-coated capsules

      iii. *Adverse effects*: Minimal adverse effects reported with oral dosing. Systemic absorption is similar to oral prednisone 2.5 mg po daily and <1 mg IV dexamethasone daily.

   b. Budesonide (Entocort EC®)

      i. *Mechanism of action*: An anti-inflammatory corticosteroid with high affinity for the glucocorticoid receptor and low systemic bioavailability due to rapid first-pass metabolism in the liver.

    ii. *Dose and administration*: 3 mg po TID or 9 mg po daily

    iii. *Adverse effects*:
- Nausea, diarrhea
- Arthralgias
- Headache
- Sinusitis, respiratory tract infection
- Cushing's syndrome
- Rare complications include immune hypersensitivity reaction, glaucoma, cataracts, increased risk of developing basal cell/squamous cell carcinoma, or malignant melanoma

8. Pentostatin (Nipent®)

  a. *Mechanism of action*: A nucleoside analog that inhibits adenosine deaminase, leading to increased levels of $2'$-deoxyadenosine $5'$-triphosphate (dATP), resulting in lymphocyte apoptosis

  b. *Dose and administration*: 1.5 mg/m^2 IV over 15–30 min on days 1–3 and 15–17. Reduce dose by 50% for ANC <1000 and/or CrCl of 30–50 mL/min, hold for ANC <500 and/or CrCl <30 mL/min.

  c. *Adverse effects*:
- i. Increased risk of infection
- ii. Cytopenias
- iii. Abdominal pain, N/V/D, anorexia
- iv. Stomatitis
- v. Headache, weakness
- vi. Transaminitis
- vii. Constitutional symptoms of fever/chills, fatigue
- viii. Rash/pruritus
- ix. Hyponatremia
- x. Acute renal failure
- xi. Microangiopathic hemolytic anemia/thrombotic thrombocytopenia purpura
- xii. Immune hypersensitivity reaction

9. Sirolimus (Rapamune®)

  a. *Mechanism of action*: Inhibits IL-2, IL-4 and IL-15 stimulated T-cell activation and proliferation, as well as inhibiting antibody production.

  b. *Dose and administration*: Load with 15 mg/m^2 po on day 1, then 5 mg/m^2 po daily × 13 days or 4–5 mg/m^2 po daily

× 14 days without a loading dose; adjust dose to maintain a trough level of 4–12 ng/mL.
c. *Adverse effects*:
  i. HUS, nephritic syndrome, renal insufficiency
  ii. Thrombotic thrombocytopenia purpura
  iii. Thromboembolism, deep vein thrombosis
  iv. Interstitial lung disease/pneumonia, pulmonary hemorrhage
  v. Hyperlipidemia
  vi. Hypertension
  vii. Rash
  viii. Abdominal pain, nausea, diarrhea, constipation
  ix. Pancytopenia
  x. Increased risk of urinary tract infections
  xi. Increased risk of developing basal cell/squamous cell carcinoma or malignant melanoma

15.9 AUTOLOGOUS GVHD

While GvHD is typically considered to be a complication of allogeneic transplant alone, an acute GvHD-like syndrome is recognized to occur in approximately 5–20% of autologous and syngeneic HSCT recipients. It is thought the incidence of autologous/syngeneic GvHD is underreported as symptoms mimic those of regimen-related toxicity.

The pathophysiology is not well understood, but is thought to be related to a failure of self-tolerance through the thymic depletion of regulatory T-cells following the conditioning regimen.

Target organs include the skin, GI tract, and liver; clinical symptoms and histopathologic findings are identical to those of allogeneic GvHD. Autologous/syngeneic GvHD most commonly affects the skin, is usually milder than allogeneic GvHD, and is often self-limiting, burning out in 1–3 weeks. Some patients, however, may require systemic steroids, and deaths have been reported, most commonly from complications of prolonged immune-suppressive therapy.

15.10 CONCLUSIONS

Only 20–40% of patients with acute GvHD will experience long-term responses to therapy, and the likelihood of response decreases as the severity of the disease increases. Of those patients with steroid-refractory disease, overall long-term survival rates fall to <20%. Patients with grade IV disease typically have <5% long-term survival.

Minimal improvement has been made in the past 10 years despite multiple new agents. Most studies have been small, and patient responses have been variable. Clinical practice relies mainly on institutional bias and provider experience. Progress in this field will depend on large multi-center clinical trials with well-defined endpoints to "standardize" responses across institutions.

References

Alousi, A., Weisdorf, D., Logan, B., Bolanos-Meade, J., Carter, S., DiFronzo, N., et al. (2009). Etanercept, mycophenlate, denileukin, or pentostatin plus corticosteroids for acute graft-versus-host disease: A randomized phase 2 trial from the Blood and Marrow Transplant Clinical Trials Network. *Blood*, 114:511–517.

Antin, J., Chen, A., Couriel, D., Ho, V., Nash, R., Weisdorf, D. (2004). Novel approaches to the therapy of steroid-resistant acute graft-versus-host disease. *Biol Blood Marrow Transplant*, 10:655–668.

Bay, J., Dhedin, N., Goerner, M., Vannier, J., Marie-Cardine, A., Stamatoullas, A., et al. (2005). Inolimomab in steroid-refractory acute graft-versus-host disease following allogeneic hematopoietic stem cell transplantation: Retrospective analysis and comparison of other interleukin-2 receptor antibodies. *Transplantation*, 80:782–788.

Bertz, H., Afting, M., Kreisel, W., Duffner, U., Greinwalkd, R., Finke, J. (1999). Feasibility and response to budesonide as topical corticosteroid therapy for acute intestinal GVHD. *Bone Marrow Transplant*, 24:1185–1189.

Bolanos-Meade, J., Jacobsohn, D., Margolis, J., Ogden, A., Wientjes, M., Byrd, J., et al. (2005). Pentostatin in steroid-refractory acute graft-versus-host disease. *J Clin Oncol*, 23:2661–2668.

Cahn, J., Klein, J., Lee, S., Milpied, N., Blaise, D., Antin, J., et al. (2005). Prospective evaluation of 2 acute graft-versus-host (GVHD) grading systems; a joint Societe Francaise de Greffe de Moelle et Therapie Cellulaire (SFGM-TC), Dana Farber Cancer Institute (DFCI) and International Transplant Registry (IBMTR) prospective study. *Blood*, 106:1495–1500.

Deeg, H. (2007). How I treat refractory acute GVHD. *Blood*, 109: 4119–4126.

Devergie, A. (2008). Graft versus host disease. In *Haematopoietic Stem Cell Transplantation: The EBMT Handbood* (pp. 218–234).

Drobyski, W., Hari, P., Keever-Taylor, C., Komorowski, R., Grossman, W. (2009). Severe autologous GVHD after hematopoietic progenitor cell transplantation for multiple myeloma. *Bone Marrow Transplant*, 43:169–177.

Duarte, R., Delgado, J., Shaw, B., Wrench, D., Ethell, M., Patch, D., et al. (2005). Histologic features of the liver biopsy predict the clinical outcome for patients with graft-versus-host disease of the liver. *Biol Blood Marrow Transplant*, 11:805–813.

Ferrera, J. (2008). Advances in the clinical management of GVHD. *Best Pract Res Clin Haematol*, 21:677–682.

Ferrera, J., Levine, J., Reddy, P., Holler, E. (2009). Graft-versus-host disease. *Lancet*, 373:1550–1561.

Funke, V., de Mederios, C., Setubal, D., Ruiz, J., Bitencourt, M., Bonfim, C., et al. (2006). Therapy for severe refractory acute graft-versus-host disease with basiliximab, a selective interleukin-2 receptor antagonist. *Bone Marrow Trasplant*, 37:961–965.

Ghez, D., Rubio, M., Maillard, N., Suarez, F., Chandesris, M., Delarue, R., et al. (2009). Rapamycin for refractory acute graft-versus-host disease. *Transplantation*, 88:1081–1087.

Greinix, H., Volc-Platzer, B., Knobler, R. (2000). Extracorporeal photochemotherapy in the treatment of severe graft-versus-host disease. *Leukemia Lymphoma*, 36:425–434.

Hess, A. (2010). Reconstitution of self-tolerance after hematopoietic stem cell transplantation. *Immunol Res*, 47:143–152.

Hoda, D., Pidala, J., Salgado-Vila, N., Kim, J., Perkins, J., Bookout, R., et al. (2009). Sirolimus for treatment of steroid-refractory acute graft-versus-host disease. *Bone Marrow Transplant*, 45:1–5.

Holmberg, L., Kikuchi, K., Gooley, T., Adams, K., Hockenbery, D., Flowers, M., et al. (2006). Gastrointestinal graft-versus-host disease in recipients of autologous hematopoietic stem cells: Incidence, risk factors and outcome. *Biol Blood Marrow Transplant*, 12:226–234.

Ibrahim, R., Abidi, M., Cronin, S., Lum, L., Al-Kadhimi, Z., Ratanatharathorn, V., et al. (2009). Nonabsorbable corticosteroids use in the treatment of gastrointestinal graft-versus-host disease. *Biol Blood Marrow Transplant*, 15:395–405.

Jacobsohn, D., Vogelsang, G. (2007). Acute graft versus host disease. *Orphanet J Rare Diseases* 2.

Johnson, M., Farmer, E. (1998). Graft-versus-host disease reactions in dermatology. *J Am Acad Dermatol*, 38:369–396.

Kim, S. (2007). Treatment options in steroid-refractory acute graft-versus-host disease following hematopoietic stem cell transplantation. *Ann Pharmacother*, 41:1436–1444.

Kuykendall, T., Smoller, B. (2003). Lack of specificity in skin biopsy specimens to assess for acute graft-versus-host disease in initial 3 weeks after bone marrow transplantation. *J Am Acad Dermatol*, 49:1081–1085.

Levine, J., Paczesny, S., Mineishi, S., Braun, T., Choi, S., Hutchinson, R., et al. (2008). Etanercept plus methylprednisolone as initial therapy for acute graft-versus-host disease. *Blood*, 111:2470–2475.

Paczesny, S., Choi, S., Ferrara, J. (2009). Acute graft-versus-host disease: New treatment strategies. *Curr Opin Hematol*, 16:427–436.

Patriarca, F., Sperotto, A., Damiani, D., Morreale, G., Bonifazi, F., Olivieri, A., et al. (2004). Infliximab treatment for steroid-refractory acute graft-versus-host disease. *Haematologica*, 89:1352–1359.

Perfetti, P., Carlier, P., Strada, P., Gualandi, F., Occhini, D., Van Lint, M., et al. (2008). Extracorporeal photopheresis for the treatment of steroid refractory acute GVHD. *Bone Marrow Transplant*, 42:609–617.

Pidala, J., Anasetti, C. (2010). Glucocorticoid-refractory acute graft-versus-host disease. *Biol Blood Marrow Transplant*, EPUB 2010 JAN 19.

Pilada, J., Kim, J., Anasetti, C. (2009). Sirolimus as primary treatment of acute graft-versus-host disease following allogeneic hematopoietic stem cell transplantation. *Biol Blood Marrow Transplant*, 15:881–885.

Pinana, J., Valcarcel, D., Martino, R., Moreno, M., Sureda, A., Briones, J., et al. (2006). Encouraging results with inolimomab (anti-IL-2 receptor) as treatment for refractory graft-versus-host disease. *Biol Blood Marrow Transplant*, 12:1135–1141.

Ross, W., Couriel, D. (2004). Colonic graft-versus-host disease. *Curr Opin Gastroenterol*, 21:64–69.

Rowlings, PA., Przepiorka, D., Klein, JP., Gale, RP., Passweg, JR., Henslee-Downey, PJ., et al. (1997). IBMTR Severity Index for grading acute graft-versus-host disease: Retrospective comparison with Glucksberg grade. *Br J Haematol*, 97:855–864.

Scarisbrick, J. (2009). Extracorporeal photopheresis: What is it and when should it be used. *Clin Exp Dermatol*, 34:757–760.

Schmidt-Hieber, M., Fietz, T., Knauf, W., Uharek, L., Hopfenmuller, W., Thiel, E., et al. (2005). Efficacy of the interleukin-2 receptor antagonist basiliximab in steroid-refractory acute graft-versus-host disease. *Br J Haematology*, 130:568–574.

Shapira, M., Resnick, I., Bitan, M., Ackerstein, A., Tsirigotis, P., Gesundheit, B., et al. (2005). Rapid responses to alefacept given to patients with steroid resistant or steroid dependent acute graft-versus-host disease: A preliminary report. *Bone Marrow Transplant*, 36:1097–1101.

Snover, D., Weisdorf, S., Ramsay, N., McGlave, P., Kersey, J. (1984). Hepatic graft versus host disease: A study of the predictive value of liver biopsy in diagnosis. *Hepatology*, 4:123–130.

Vogelsang, G., Lee, L., Bensen-Kennedy, D. (2003). Pathogenesis and treatment of graft-versus-host disease after bone marrow transplant. *Annu Rev Med*, 54:29–52.

CHAPTER 16
Chronic Graft-Versus-Host Disease

Richard T. Maziarz and Farnoush Abar

Chronic graft-versus-host disease (cGvHD) is the single major factor influencing long-term outcome and quality of life after allogeneic transplantation. However, the presence of cGvHD has been linked to decrease in relapse rate of patients with CML, ALL, and AML. In a recent CIBMTR/NMDP analysis of ~3500 transplant patients with cGvHD, risk of relapse was reduced by 50%. Traditionally, cGvHD has been defined as occurring after day +100, this entity has been documented as early as 50 days to years after the transplant procedure. Chronic GvHD can emerge during or immediately following taper of immune suppressive agents or may occur as part of a continuous spectrum merging acute GvHD into cGvHD (progressive GvHD). It may occur suddenly after a "quiescent" period of time following resolution of previous GvHD or "de novo" in a patient who has had no previous GvHD. Chronic GvHD is an alloimmune process (donor versus recipient) that results in alloantibody formation as well as anti-host T-cell responses and may involve a single or multi-organ system focus.

The syndrome of cGvHD has features resembling various autoimmune disorders including scleroderma, Sjogren's syndrome, membranous glomerulonephritis, and immune cytopenias from which much of our current therapy has been based.

16.1 INCIDENCE AND PROGNOSIS
The incidence of cGvHD can range from 30 to 90% depending on risk factors. Skin involvement is common. Patients with traditionally staged using the original Fred Hutchinson

R.T. Maziarz, S. Slater (eds.), *Blood and Marrow Transplant Handbook*, DOI 10.1007/978-1-4419-7506-5_16, © Springer Science+Business Media, LLC 2011

Cancer Research Center definition of "limited disease" (localized involvement, hepatic dysfunction, or both) have a more favorable prognosis. Those who have "extensive disease" (generalized skin involvement, localized skin + hepatic dysfunction + ocular involvement or salivary gland involvement, or any other target organ), especially disease involving multiple body systems/organs, have a more unrelenting and unfavorable disease course. If the patient can survive, often tolerance will occur and the patient may improve, thus allowing the cGvHD to eventually "burn itself out." After bone marrow transplant procedures, 80% of patients can be withdrawn from immune suppression 2–3 years from diagnosis of cGvHD. Recent analyses identified that ∼50% of cGvHD patients are not able to be weaned from immune-suppressive therapy by 5 years after peripheral blood stem cell transplant (Fig. 16.1).

Other poor prognostic indicators include progressive GvHD (acute progressing directly to chronic) with associated increased nonrelapse mortality, thrombocytopenia that persists to day +100 (30–40% 5-year survival compared to 80% 5-year survival for patients with platelet counts >100,000), and elevated serum bilirubin.

A cGvHD staging system from Johns Hopkins Medical Center assesses three factors: extensive skin involvement (>50% body surface area), thrombocytopenia (platelets <100,000/mm^3), and progressive type onset. Projected survival ranged

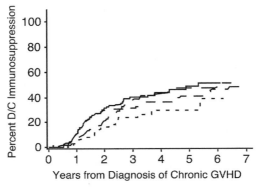

FIG. 16.1. Time to immune suppression withdrawal after PBSC transplantation. Stewart et al., Blood, 2004, © American Society of Hematology

between 9% and 84% at 3 years, based on the number of indicators identified in the patient population.

Finally, a CIBMTR analysis of newly diagnosed cGvHD identified that performance status, diarrhea, and weight loss were also factors that contribute to enhanced nonrelapse mortality.

Two years after allogeneic transplant, cGvHD becomes the greatest risk to overall survival.

16.2 RISK FACTORS

1. Previous acute GvHD
2. Age of recipient (GvHD increases with recipient's age)
3. Parous female donor
4. Use of multiple-transfused donor
5. Use of allogeneic blood stem cells instead of bone marrow
6. Mismatched donor graft
7. History of acute inflammation (sunburn, toxic epidermal necrolysis, Stevens Johnson syndrome, etc.)
8. CMV seropositivity
9. Sex-mismatched donor graft
10. DLI utilization
11. Unrelated donor transplantation

16.3 STIGMATA/CLINICAL FEATURES OF CGVHD

Historically, determination of cGvHD was based on primary presentation and was limited in scope. With recognition that chronic GvHD is a multi-organ process that can be a relenting/relapsing disorder, new detailed diagnostic criteria have been agreed upon by consensus. An adaptation of these consensus criteria (see Filopovich et al., 2005) for signs and symptoms of cGvHD is provided in Table 16.1.

16.4 DIAGNOSIS AND GRADING

As previously described, grading has historically been classified based on primary presentation and relatively limited in the detail of the assessment. An updated approach to the global assessment of cGvHD diagnosis and severity became necessary. This approach was found to be more clinically suitable and appropriate for use as inclusion criteria in therapeutic clinical trials or as indications for systemic immunosuppressive

TABLE 16.1. Stigmata and clinical features of cGvHD

Organ or site	Diagnostic (adequate for the diagnosis of cGvHD)	Distinctive (seen in cGvHD but not aGvHD; insufficient to establish cGvHD diagnosis)	Other features (cannot be used to establish a diagnosis)	Common (seen with aGvHD and cGvHD)
Skin	Poikiloderma Lichen-type features Sclerotic features Morphea-like features Lichen-sclerosis	Vitiligo	Sweat impairment Ichtyosis Keratosis pilaris Decreased pigmentation Increased pigmentation	Erythema Maculopapular rash Pruritus
Nails		Dystrophy Longitudinal ridging, splitting, brittleness Onycholysis Pterygium Destruction (usually symmetric, affects most nails)		
Scalp and body hair		New alopecia (after recovery from chemoradiotherapy), scarring and nonscarring alopecia; scaling, papulosquamous lesions Loss of body hair, typically patchy (including eyelashes, eyebrows)	Thinning scalp hair, coarse or dull (not due to endocrine or other causes) Premature gray hair	

TABLE 16.1. *(Continued)*

Organ or site	Diagnostic (adequate for the diagnosis of cGvHD)	Distinctive (seen in cGvHD but not aGvHD; insufficient to establish cGvHD diagnosis)	Other features (cannot be used to establish a diagnosis)	Common (seen with aGvHD and cGvHD)
Mouth	Lichen-type features Hyperkeratotic plaques Sclerosis with decreased range of motion	Xerostomia Mucocele Mucosal atrophy Ulcers Pseudomembranes		Gingivitis Mucositis Erythema Pain
Eyes		New onset dry, gritty, or painful eyes Cicatricial conjunctivitis Keratoconjunctivitis sicca Corneal ulceration	Excessive aqueous tearing Photophobia Periorbital hyperpigmentation Blepharitis	
Genitalia	Lichen-type features Vaginal strictures or stenosis	Ulcers Fissures Erosion		

TABLE 16.1. (*Continued*)

Organ or site	Diagnostic (adequate for the diagnosis of cGvHD)	Distinctive (seen in cGvHD but not aGvHD; insufficient to establish cGvHD diagnosis)	Other features (cannot be used to establish a diagnosis)	Common (seen with aGvHD and cGvHD)
GI Tract	Esophageal webbing Strictures or stenosis in the upper-third of the esophagus		Pancreatic insufficiency	Anorexia Nausea Vomiting Diarrhea Weight loss
Liver				Failure to thrive Total bilirubin, alk phos > 2× ULN ALT or AST >2× ULN
Lung	Bronchiolitis obliterans diagnosed with lung biopsy	Bronchiolitis obliterans diagnosed with PFTs and radiology		BOOP
Muscles Fascia Joints	Fasciitis Joint stiffness of contractures secondary to sclerosis	Myositis or polymyositis (proximal muscle weakness; myalgia is uncommon)	Edema Muscle cramps Arthralgia or arthritis	

TABLE 16.1. (*Continued*)

Organ or site	Diagnostic (adequate for the diagnosis of cGvHD)	Distinctive (seen in cGvHD but not aGvHD; insufficient to establish cGvHD diagnosis)	Other features (cannot be used to establish a diagnosis)	Common (seen with aGvHD and cGvHD)
Hematopoietic			Thrombocytopenia	
			Eosinophilia	
			Lymphopenia	
			Hypo- or hyper gammaglobulinemia	
			Autoantibodies (also AIHA, ITP)	
Other			Pericardial or pleural effusions	
			Ascites	
			Peripheral neuropathy	
			Nephrotic syndrome	
			Myasthenia gravis	
			Cardiac conduction abnormality or cardiomyopathy	

therapy. In 2005, the National Institutes of Health conducted a Consensus Development Project for determining the criteria for Clinical Trial Development for cGvHD. The focus was on how to optimize the design of future clinical trials, diagnosis and staging, biomarker assessment, establishment of systematic histopathology grading, determination of distinct response criteria, and identification of uniform ancillary therapy and supportive care recommendations.

Now as a more universally accepted and as a consequence of the NIH conference, the current consensus recommends that the diagnosis of cGvHD should require at least one diagnostic manifestation of cGvHD or at least two distinctive manifestations (one confirmed by lab testing, radiology, or biopsy) [see Table 16.1]. Infection and other diagnoses may confound the differential diagnosis of cGvHD and must be excluded. Biopsy is often helpful, but not always possible.

Additionally, a clinical scoring system was developed to assist in the evaluation of individual organs, as well as global assessment of the impact of the disease to the individual. Based on this assessment, systemic therapy could then be recommended for patients who meet moderate to severe global severity.

This updated scoring system, based on the clinical impact of cGvHD on the patient's performance status, is shown in Table 16.2.

16.5 MONITORING

Serial monitoring of all organ systems affected by cGvHD is recommended and should be performed at least annually for up to 5 years after transplant. The evaluation should include medical, psychosocial, nutritional, and developmental assessments including Tanner scoring in children and adolescents. These measures allow for instituting preventive and early treatment measures.

Suggested monitoring studies include:

1. Complete blood cell counts with differential (every 1–6 months)
2. Chemistry panel including renal and liver function tests (every 1–6 months)
3. Therapeutic drug monitoring (every 1–6 months)
4. IgG level (every 1–6 months until normal without need for replacement)

TABLE 16.2. NIH cGHVD organ-specific staging form

	Score 0	Score 1	Score 2	Score 3
Performance score KPS ECOG LPS	☐ Asymptomatic and fully active (ECOG 0; KPS or LPS 100%)	☐ Symptomatic, fully ambulatory, restricted only in physically strenuous activity (ECOG 1, KPS or LPS 80–90%)	☐ Symptomatic, ambulatory, capable of self-care, >50% of waking hours out of bed (ECOG 2, KPS or LPS 60–70%)	☐ Symptomatic, limited self-care, >50% of waking hours in bed (ECOG 3–4, KPS or LPS <60%)
SKIN Clinical features	☐ No symptoms with no or minimal distinct signs	☐ <18% BSA with disease signs but NO sclerotic features	☐ 19–50% BSA OR superficial sclerotic features "not hidebound" (able to pinch)	☐ >50% BSA OR deep sclerotic features "hidebound" (unable to pinch) OR interference with ADL due to impaired mobility, ulceration or severe pruritus
☐ Maculopapular rash ☐ Lichen-type features ☐ Papulosquamous or ichthyosis ☐ Hyperpigmentation				

TABLE 16.2. (*Continued*)

	Score 0	Score 1	Score 2	Score 3
☐ Hypopigmentation ☐ Keratosis pilaris ☐ Erythema ☐ Erythroderma ☐ Poikiloderma ☐ Sclerotic features ☐ Pruritus ☐ Hair ☐ Nails				
%BSA involved MOUTH	☐ No symptoms with no or minimal distinct signs	☐ Mild symptoms with disease signs, but not limiting oral intake significantly	☐ Moderate symptoms with signs with partial limitation of oral intake	☐ Severe symptoms with disease signs on examination with major limitation of oral intake
EYES	☐ No symptoms	☐ Mild dry eye symptoms not affecting ADL (requiring eye drops ≤3× per day) OR symptomatic signs of sicca keratitis	☐ Moderate dry eye symptoms partially affecting ADL (requiring drops >3× per day or punctal plugs), WITHOUT vision impairment	☐ Severe dry eye symptoms significantly affecting ADL (special eyewear to relieve pain) OR unable to work due to
Mean tear test (mm): ☐ >10 ☐ 6–10 ☐ ≤5 ☐ Not done				

TABLE 16.2. (*Continued*)

	Score 0	Score 1	Score 2	Score 3
				ocular symptoms OR loss of vision caused by pseudomembranes or corneal ulceration
GI TRACT	□ No symptoms	□ ≤ Symptoms such as dysphagia, anorexia, nausea, vomiting, abdominal pain, or diarrhea without significant weight loss (<5%)	□ Symptoms associated with mild to moderate weight loss (5–15%)	□ Symptoms associated with significant weight loss >15%, requires nutritional supplement for most calorie needs OR esophageal dilation
LIVER	□ Normal LFTs	□ Bilirubin, AP, AST, or ALT <2 × ULN	□ Bilirubin >3 mg/dL or bili, enzymes 2–5 × ULN	□ Bili or enzymes >5 × ULN

TABLE 16.2. (Continued)

	Score 0	Score 1	Score 2	Score 3
LUNGS	☐ No symptoms ☐ FEV1/FVC ratio <0.75 OR FEV1 of 51–75%, without distinct findings of bronchiolitis obliterans (BO) on HRCT	☐ Mild symptoms (dyspnea with stair climbing) ☐ FEV1/FVC ratio <0.75 OR FEV1 of 51–75% WITH mild distinct findings of BO on HRCT	☐ Moderate symptoms (dyspnea with level walking) ☐ FEV1/FVC ratio <0.75 OR FEV1 of 35–50% WITH distinct findings of BO on HRCT	☐ Severe symptoms (dyspnea at rest; requiring 02) ☐ FEV1/FVC ratio of <0.75 OR FEV1 ≤34% WITH distinct findings of BO on HRCT
JOINTS AND FASCIA	☐ No symptoms	☐ Mild tightness of arms or legs, normal or mild decreased ROM AND not affecting ADL	☐ Tightness of arms or legs or joint contractures erythema thought due to fasciitis, moderate decreased ROM *AND* mild to moderate limitation of ADL	☐ Contractures WITH significant decrease of ROM AND significant limitation of ADL (unable to tie shoes, button shirts, dress self, etc.)

TABLE 16.2. (*Continued*)

	Score 0	Score 1	Score 2	Score 3
GENITAL TRACT	☐ No symptoms with no or minimal distinct signs on examination	☐ Symptomatic with mild distinct signs on exam AND no effect on coitus and minimal discomfort with GYN exam	☐ Symptomatic with distinct signs on exam AND with mild dyspareunia or discomfort with GYN Exam	☐ Symptomatic WITH advanced signs (stricture, labia agglutination, or severe ulceration) AND severe pain with coitus or inability to insert vaginal speculum
☐ Weight loss ☐ BO (lungs)	☐ Eosinophilia ≥500/μL	☐ Progressive onset ☐ Disabling contractures		
☐ Malabsorption ☐ BOOP (lungs) ☐ Esophageal stricture or web	☐ Fasciitis ☐ Plts <100,000 μL ☐ Myositis ☐ Serositis	☐ None		

Filipovich, et al., 2005

5. Lipid profile (every 6–12 months, especially while on treatment with systemic steroids or sirolimus)
6. Iron indices (every 6–12 months if history of iron overload or red blood cell transfusions requirement)
7. Pulmonary function tests (every 3–12 months)
8. Endocrine function evaluation including thyroid function tests, testosterone level (every 12 months)
9. Bone densitometry, calcium levels, 25-OH vitamin D (every 12 months)

16.6 THERAPY

Symptomatic mild cGvHD can often be managed with local therapy alone, e.g., topical corticosteroids. However, in patients with disease involving three or more organs or with a score of ≥ 2 in any single organ, systemic immunosuppression may be considered. Organ system-specific preventive measures and ancillary treatments are a critical part of cGvHD management and can decrease the need for high dose and/or prolonged systemic treatment.

Systemic treatment strategies include:

1. Prednisone: 1 mg/kg po daily, then taper as tolerated. This dose is usually continued for a minimum of 1–2 weeks prior to initiation of taper. Some centers advocate an every other day dosing schedule.
2. Cyclosporine: Dose adjusted to maintain a therapeutic target level of 100–150. Used in combination with prednisone improves patients' survival as compared with prednisone alone.
3. Mycophenolate mofetil (Cellcept®): 0.5–1.5 gm po BID; long-term use has been tolerated, but recent data suggest that some patients with new diagnosis of cGvHD will have enhanced risk of mortality when receiving primary treatment with mycophenolate in combination with calcineurin inhibitors and steroids (Martin et al., 2009)
4. Tacrolimus (FK 506, Prograf®): Initially, 0.03–0.05 mg/kg/day CI or 0.075–0.15 mg/kg po every 12 h. Adjust dose as necessary to maintain therapeutic drug level of 5–10.
5. Sirolimus (Rapamune®): Loading dose of 4 mg po × 1 followed by 1–2 mg po once daily. Adjust dose as necessary to maintain therapeutic drug level of 6–12. Contraindicated to be given with voriconazole.

6. Acetretin (Soriatane®): Starting dose of 10 mg po daily. Increase as tolerated to a maximum dosing of 40 mg po daily. Can be effective in cutaneous cGvHD, but needs to be used with caution.
7. Plaquenil: 3.5–5.0 mg/kg/day po in 2–3 divided doses (do not exceed 400 mg/day)
8. Extracorporeal photopheresis: Well-tolerated procedure with unclear mechanism of action although is felt to be associated with expansion of regulatory T-cell populations (Treg) that can modulate signs and symptoms. Varying schedules have been used.
   a. Our current institutional approach includes photopheresis for two consecutive days, repeated every 2 weeks for a total of 12 weeks. Then, two consecutive days of treatment every month for 6 months.
   b. Line placement and maintaining integrity of central lines can be difficult in patients with hide-like sclerodermatous changes.
   c. Payer support for these procedures is usually available, but there can be variable funding for long-term central line maintenance.
9. Other treatments that have been used with some reported response, either anecdotally or in phase 2 trials:
   a. Pentostatin
   b. Rituximab
   c. Clofazamine
   d. Thalidomide
   e. Inflixomab
   f. Etanercept
   g. PUVA
   h. Imatinib mesylate
   i. Total nodal irradiation

Organ-specific therapies are outlined in Table 16.3. Some practical and clinical guidelines for management of the cGvHD patient include:

1. Skin:
   a. Steroid creams/ointments
      i. From the neck down: Start with mid-strength topical steroids (e.g., triamcinolone 0.1% cream or ointment), may proceed to higher potency steroids (e.g., fluocinonide 0.05% cream or ointment)
      ii. Face, axillae, and groin: Lower-potency steroids (hydrocortisone 1–2.5%, desonide 0.05%)

TABLE 16.3. Organ-specific management for cGvHD (adapted from Couriel, BBMT, 2006)

Ancillary therapy and supportive care interventions

Organ	Prevention	Treatment
Skin and appendages	Photoprotection Surveillance for malignancy	Intact skin – topical emollients, corticosteroids, antipruritic agents, and others (e.g., psoralen–UV-A, calcineurin inhibitors). Erosions/ulcerations – Microbiologic cultures, topical antimicrobials, protective films or other dressings, debridement, hyperbaric oxygen, wound care specialist consultation
Mouth and oral cavity	Maintain good oral hygiene. Routine dental cleaning Endocarditis prophylaxis	Topical corticosteroids; therapy for xerostomia
Eyes	Photoprotection Surveillance for infection, cataract formation, and increased intraocular pressure	Artificial tears, topical corticosteroids or cyclosporine, punctal occlusion, humidified environment, occlusive eye wear, moisture chamber eyeglasses, cevimeline, pilocarpine, tarsorraphy, gas-permeable scleral contact lens, topical antimicrobials, doxycycline, autologous serum drops
Lung	Surveillance for infection (*Pneumocystis jiroveci*, viral, fungal, bacterial) Prevent aspiration/gastroesophageal reflux	Bronchodilators, supplementary oxygen, Azithromycin, pulmonary rehabilitation

TABLE 16.3. (*Continued*)

Ancillary therapy and supportive care interventions

Organ	Prevention	Treatment
Vulva and vagina	Early gynecologic consultation Surveillance for estrogen deficiency, infection (herpes simplex virus, human papilloma virus, yeast, bacteria), malignancy	Water-based lubricants, topical estrogens, topical steroids or calcineurin inhibitors, dilators, surgery for synechiae/obliteration
Gastrointestinal tract and liver	Surveillance for infection (viral, fungal)	Dietary modification, enzyme supplementation for malabsorption, gastroesophageal reflux management, esophageal dilatation, ursodeoxycholic acid (liver)
Neurologic	Calcineurin drug-level monitoring Seizure prophylaxis including blood pressure control, electrolyte replacement, anticonvulsants	Occupational and physical therapies, treatment of neuropathic syndromes with tricyclic antidepressants, selective serotonin reuptake inhibitors, or anticonvulsants

TABLE 16.3. (Continued)

Ancillary therapy and supportive care interventions

Organ	Prevention	Treatment
Musculoskeletal	Surveillance for decreased range of motion, bone densitometry, calcium and 25-OH vitamin D levels Calcium, vitamin D, bisphosphonates Physical therapy massage	Physical therapy, massage, bisphosphonates
Immunologic and infectious disease	Surveillance for infection (cytomegalovirus, parvovirus) Immunoglobulin replacement based on levels (Chapters 8, 13) Prophylaxis against *Pneumocystis jiroveci*, varicella zoster virus, and encapsulated bacteria (Chapters 8, 13) Immunizations based on guideline of the Centers for Disease Control (Chapters 8, 13) Immune reconstitution analysis (Chapter 26)	Empiric parenteral broad-spectrum antibacterial coverage for fever (Chapter 14)

      iii. Emollients: can be used after the application of steroids. Note that emollients are occlusive and may increase the potency of steroids.

      iv. Occlusive wraps: after application of topical agent, simple maneuvers such as wearing gloves or socks or wrapping with plastic wrap for set time periods can enhance steroid delivery

  b. Antipruritics:

      i. Topical: Hydrocortisone/pramoxine or menthol-based creams/lotions.

      ii. Systemic: Antihistamines (e.g., diphenhydramine, hydroxyzine, ranitidine) or the tricyclic agent doxepin

  c. Psoralen with UV-A, UV-A1 (340–400 nm), UV-B, or narrowband UV-B (311–313 nm),

      i. Better for nonsclerotic lesions

      ii. Phototherapy schedule is typically 2–3 times per week

      iii. Associated with an increased risk of skin cancer. Hence, history of skin cancer or photosensitivity may be a contraindication

  d. Topical calcineurin inhibitors (e.g., tacrolimus).

  e. Topical bleaching agents (hydroquinone 4.0% cream)

      i. For treatment of post-inflammatory hyperpigmentation

      ii. Should not be should in setting of active disease

  f. If ulceration is present, tissue culture should rule out infection

  g. In denuded skin, wound dressings improve regeneration/repair of epithelium

      i. May use ± topical antimicrobials such as mupirocin ointment or silver-containing products

      ii. Do not use high-potency steroid under dressing, as it can potentiate the strength of steroid.

2. Mouth and oral cavity

  a. Topical steroid

      i. Standard dexamethasone (5 mg diluted in 15 mL of water) rinse: swished in the mouth for 4–6 min and then expelled without swallowing, 4–6 times per day

      ii. High-potency corticosteroid gel or ointment (fluocinonide, clobetasol, or betamethasone dipropionate) applied locally.

>
> iii. Note high-potency steroids can cause irreversible atrophy when applied to the vermillion border of the lips
> iv. Monitor for oral candidiasis
> b. Tacrolimus ointment
> c. Topical analgesia such as viscous lidocaine when symptomatic mucosal GvHD affecting oral intake and/or speech
> d. Xerostomia: encourage water sipping, use of salivary stimulants (sugar-free gum and candy), saliva substitutes. Note dry mouth increases the risk of tooth decay, hence topical fluorides should be used
> e. Sialogogue therapy with cholinergic agonists (cevimeline, pilocarpine) to increase salivary secretion (contraindications include glaucoma, heart disease, or asthma)
> f. Routine dental care, consider antibiotic prophylaxis in patients with delayed immune reconstitution, neutropenia
> 3. Eyes:
> a. Defined by keratoconjunctivitis sicca (KCS) syndrome with tear production averaging ≤5 mm (defined by Schirmer test) and clinical signs of keratitis
> b. Infectious keratitis must be ruled out
> c. Mild artificial tears, viscous ointment (Lacrilube®) at bedtime, flax seed oil
> d. Moderate/severe
>> i. Steroid drops (must be monitored for toxicities such as increased intraocular pressure, cataract formation, and silent infectious keratitis)
>> ii. Cyclosporine drops
>> iii. Lacrimal plugs if > hourly use of artificial tears
>> iv. Barrier eyeglasses (diminishes environmental effects, e.g., wind convection)
>> iv. Minimize evaporation and maximize the output of outer oil layer of the tear film (warm compresses, Doxycycline if rosacea blepharitis/meibomitis
>> v. Oral agents such as pilocarpine and cevimeline (these have been shown to improve sicca symptoms in patients with Sjögren syndrome, contraindications include glaucoma, heart disease, and asthma.)
>> vi. Surgical approaches (punctal occlusion, superficial debridement of filamentary keratitis, partial tarsorrhaphy)

       vii. Other approaches utilized, but less generally available, include autologous serum eye drops, gas-permeable contact lens (e.g., Boston scleral lens prosthesis®).

4. Lung:
   a. Bronchodilators and steroid inhalers are the mainstay of treatment
   b. Evaluate and treat for:
      i. Gastroesophageal reflux disease and/or silent pulmonary aspiration
   c. Monitor obstructive/restrictive changes on PFTs q 3 months
      i. Note: DL_{CO} should be corrected for hemoglobin but not for alveolar volume, and lung volumes should be preferentially measured with body plethysmography and not with a gas-based method.
   d. Pulmonary rehabilitation programs
   e. Prophylactic immunoglobulin infusions do not prevent bronchiolitis obliterans
   f. Chronic azithromycin treatment may be beneficial in bronchiolitis obliterans by reducing inflammatory process

5. Gastrointestinal tract:
   a. Odynophagia and dysphagia
      i. Endoscopic evaluation for esophageal webs, rings, strictures with recognition that esophageal dilation has risk of perforation
   b. Diarrhea
      i. GvHD: nonabsorbable steroids
      ii. Assess for infection e.g., *Clostridium difficile* toxin screen, cytomegalovirus (CMV) cultures, endoscopy (because CMV can cause colitis without antigenemia)
   c. Assess lactose intolerance
   d. Pancreatic insufficiency requiring pancreatic enzyme supplementation
   e. Review medication schedule for drug-induced diarrhea, e.g., magnesium oxide and MMF
   f. Weight loss/malnutrition workup usually identifies multifactorial etiology including dysphagia, malabsorption, pancreatic enzyme deficiency, depression

6. Hepatic
   a. Assessment of abnormal liver function tests
      i. rule out gallbladder disease, liver abscess, infiltration by imaging

        ii. Consider evaluation and treatment of iron overload

        iii. Ursodeoxycholic acid can help to improve biochemical abnormalities and pruritus

7. Vaginal/vulvar:
   a. Rule out infectious etiology (bacterial, human papilloma virus, HSV, yeast)
   b. Determine if 2° estrogen deficiency with replacement
   c. Topical hydrocortisone (e.g., high vaginal application of hydrocortisone acetate 100 mg/d; mucoadherent rectal foam 1 g daily for 4–6 weeks, followed by serial reduction in dose frequency according to response)
   d. Topical cyclosporine (e.g., cyclosporine oral solution 100 mg/mL, 1 mL in 20 mL normal saline high vaginal installation for 15 min daily for 4–6 weeks, followed by serial reduction in dose frequency according to response)
   e. Vaginal dilatation once to twice daily for established vaginal stenosis, and then when adequate vaginal capacity is achieved, can continue 2× weekly. Dilatation can be achieved with commercially available dilators, intercourse, or self digital examination.

8. Neurologic
   a. Consider VZV reactivation as etiology of neuropathy
   b. Treat painful neuropathy with, e.g., gabapentin, pregabalin, selective serotonin reuptake inhibitors, and anticonvulsants, NOT narcotics

9. Musculoskeletal
   a. Fasciitis, sclerotic contractures, and limitation in the range of motion: aggressive physical therapy with focus on ROM exercises, stretching, yoga, massage
   b. Steroid-induced myopathy can be managed with physical therapy and steroid withdrawal
   c. Osteoporosis - Calcium/VitD,bisphosphonates (Chapter 13)

10. Immunologic/infectious disease
    a. Antibacterial prophylaxis: required for encapsulated bacteria protection, in particular *Streptococcus pneumoniae*, but also *Haemophilus influenzae*, and *Neisseria meningitides* in all patients with cGvHD as long as on systemic immunosuppressive. Penicillin VK or erythromycin/ azithromycin are commonly used
    b. Vaccination (See Chapter 13 for details)
    c. Intravenous immunoglobulin (See Chapter 13 for details)

16.7 FOLLOW-UP

1. Multi-organ system follow-up every 1–2 months with consistent evaluator
2. Extended protective precautions
3. Prompt evaluation of fever
4. The ultimate goal of treatment is to achieve cure, i.e., immunologic tolerance of the cGvHD, which is manifest as improvement of all symptoms and signs of the disorder. However, it remains sobering that the majority of patients will require long-term immune suppression. A recent phase 3 randomized trial comparing steroids with calcineurin inhibitors compared to steroids with calcineurin inhibitors and mycophenolate demonstrated that there was no difference in the number of patients who were completely tapered from immune suppression at 2 years, and that in both arms approximately 80% of patients remained on treatment at this time point (Martin et al., 2009). These data support the need for established criteria for diagnosis and as well for determining response. Additionally, these data support the importance of patient self-reporting symptomatology for determination of quality-of-life assessments.

References

Akpek, G., Lee, S., Flowers, M., Pavletic, S., Arora, M., Lee, S., et al. (2003). Performance of a new clinical graft-versus-host disease: A multicenter study. *Blood*, 102:802–809.

Cosar, C.B., Cohen, E.J., Rapuano, C.J., et al. (2001). Tarsorrhaphy: Clinical experience from a cornea practice. *Cornea*, 20:787–791.

Couriel, D., Carpenter, P.A., Cutler, C., Bolaños-Meade, J., Treiste, Sr N., Gea-Banacloche, J., et al. (2006). Ancillary therapy and supportive care of chronic graft-versus-host disease: National Institutes of Health Consensus Development Project on Criteria for Clinical Trials in Chronic Graft-versus-Host Disease: V. Ancillary Therapy and Supportive Care Working Group Report. *Biol Blood Marrow Transplant*, 12:375–396.

Elad, S., Or, R., Resnick, I., Shapira, M.Y. (2003). Topical tacrolimus-a novel treatment alternative for cutaneous chronic graft-versus-host disease. *Transpl Int*, 16:665–670.

Filipovich, A., Weisdorf, D., Pavletic, S., Socie, G., Wingard, J., Lee, S., et. at. (2005). National institutes of health consensus development project on criteria for clinical trials in chronic graft-versus-host disease: I. Diagnosis and staging working group report. *Biol Blood Marrow Transplant*, 12:945–955.

Grundmann-Kollmann, M., Martin, H., Ludwig, R., et al. (2002). Narrowband UV-B phototherapy in the treatment of cutaneous graft versus host disease. *Transplantation*, 74:1631–1634.

Kerstjens, H.A., Brand, P.L., Hughes, M.D., et al. (1992). A comparison of bronchodilator therapy with or without inhaled corticosteroid therapy for obstructive airways disease. Dutch chronic non-specific lung disease study group. *N Engl J Med*, 327:1413–1419.

Kojima, T., Ishida, R., Dogru, M., et al. (2005). The effect of autologous serum eyedrops in the treatment of severe dry eye disease: A prospective randomized case-control study. *Am J Ophthalmol*, 139:242–246.

Martin, P., Storer, B., Rowley, S., Flowers, M., Lee, S., Carpenter, P., et al. (2009). Evaluation of mycophenolate mofetil for initial treatment of chronic graft-versus-host disease. *Blood*, 113:5074–5082.

Ogawa, Y., Okamoto, S., Mori, T., et al. (2003). Autologous serum eyedrops for the treatment of severe dry eye in patients with chronic graft-versus-host disease. *Bone Marrow Transplant*, 31:579–583.

Pavletic, S., Martin, P., Lee, S., Mitchell, S., Jacobsen, D., Cowen, E., et al. (2006). Measuring therapeutic response in chronic graft-versus-host disease: National Institutes of Health Development Project on Criteria for Clinical Trials in Chronic Graft-versus-Host Disease: IV. Response Criteria Working Group Report. *Biol Blood Marrow Transplant*, 12:252–266.

Robinson, M.R., Lee, S.S., Rubin, B.I., et al. (2004). Topical corticosteroid therapy for cicatricial conjunctivitis associated with chronic graft-versus-host disease. *Bone Marrow Transplant*, 33:1031–1035.

Rosenthal, P., Cotter, J.M., Baum, J. (2000). Treatment of persistent corneal epithelial defect with extended wear of a fluid-ventilated gas-permeable scleral contact lens. *Am J Ophthalmol*, 130:33–41.

Sall, K., Stevenson, O.D., Mundorf, T.K., Reis, B.L. (2000). Two multicenter, randomized studies of the efficacy and safety of cyclosporine ophthalmic emulsion in moderate to severe dry eye disease. CsA Phase 3 study group. *Ophthalmology*, 107:631–639.

Stewart, B., Storer, B., Storek, J., Deeg, H., Storb, R., Hansen, J., et al. (2004). Duration of immunosuppressive treatment for chronic graft-versus-host disease. *Blood*, 104:3501–3506.

Sullivan, K.M. (1996). Immunomodulation in allogeneic marrow transplantation: Use of intravenous immune globulin to suppress acute graft-versus-host disease. *Clin Exp Immunol*, 104(suppl 1):43–48.

Wetzig, T., Sticherling, M., Simon, J.C., Hegenbart, U., Niederwieser, D., Al-Ali, H.K. (2005). Medium dose long-wavelength ultravioletA (UVA1) phototherapy for the treatment of acute and chronic graft-versus-host disease of the skin. *Bone Marrow Transplant*, 35:515–519.

Yates, B., Murphy, D.M., Forrest, I.A., Ward, C., Rutherford, R.M., Fisher, A.J., Lordan, J.L., Dark JH, Corris, P.A. (2005). Azithromycin reverses airflow obstruction in established bronchiolitis obliterans syndrome. *Am J Respir Crit Care Med*, 172:772–775.

CHAPTER 17
Oral Complications

Kimberly Brennan Tyler

Mucositis is reported as the side effect that most negatively affects the quality of life in patients receiving cancer treatment. It is a consequence of cancer treatment that results in tissue damage manifested by erythema, edema, and ulceration of the gastrointestinal mucosa, disrupting the protective barrier. It is typically noted post-transplant and continues until the healing effects of engraftment, although one may also see similar mucosal changes associated with graft-versus-host disease (GvHD) or infection.

17.1 PATHOPHYSIOLOGY
Mucositis is the consequence of a variety of pathophysiologic processes occurring in conjunction with multiple cytokine releases, with resulting damage of the epithelial surfaces and subsequent disruption of the integrity of the epithelial layer. Due to the direct chemotherapeutic effect on epithelial tissues, there can be significant delay in repair of the damaged tissues, which further potentiates the effects of the inflammatory process. The epithelial lining is then at a greater risk for colonization of and invasion by various microorganisms. In HSCT patients, as a consequence of dose escalation of chemoradiotherapy, increased tissue damage is anticipated.

17.2 RISK FACTORS
1. Conditioning regimen
2. Medications that cause xerostomia and decrease salivation (opiates, diuretics, etc.)

R.T. Maziarz, S. Slater (eds.), *Blood and Marrow Transplant Handbook*, DOI 10.1007/978-1-4419-7506-5_17, © Springer Science+Business Media, LLC 2011

3. Prolonged antimicrobial usage
4. Prolonged hospitalization
5. Prolonged myelosuppression
6. History of mucositis with previous treatment cycles
7. Body mass index (>25 increases risk of OM)
8. Conditioning regimens (TBI, melphalan)
9. GvHD prophylaxis (calcineurin inhibitor)
10. Emesis
11. Poor oral health and hygiene
12. Poor nutritional status
13. Tobacco and alcohol use
14. Infectious disease exposures (e.g., Herpes simplex)
15. GvHD
16. Mouth breathing

17.3 PROPHYLAXIS

1. Oral hygiene prior to admission
   a. Brushing with fluoride toothpaste BID and flossing daily
   b. Use foam toothbrush if painful mucositis precludes use of a regular toothbrush, or once platelet count falls below 50,000/μL. Daily flossing if atraumatic and platelet count is >50,000/μL.
   c. Chlorhexidine 0.12% contains alcohol and should only be used to minimize bacterial colonization prior to signs of OM. Chlorhexidine 0.12% aqueous alcohol-free solution is available by prescription through a dentist's office.
   d. Pre-transplant dental evaluation and cleaning by a dentist with experience working with stem cell transplant patients.
      i. All sources of dental infection should be preferentially corrected prior to conditioning. Badly decayed teeth/dental carries may require extraction.
      ii. Patients receiving IV bisphosphonates require special consideration and conservative management of dental problems to reduce the risk of osteonecrosis of the jaw
      iii. Mucosa should be healed 10–14 days prior to conditioning regimen
   e. Low-level laser therapy to reduce plaques before HSCT if available.
   f. Orthodontic bands should be removed
   g. Avoid the use of other dental appliances unless they have been evaluated and approved prior to transplant.

   h. Avoid alcohol and tobacco

2. Oral hygiene during transplant

   a. Ongoing oral assessment using validated staging tool (see Table 17.1).

   b. Encourage the patient to communicate symptoms in a timely manner for prompt initiation of therapy.

   c. Palifermin (Kepivance®) 60 mcg/kg/day on 3 consecutive days, with the last dose given no less than 24 h prior to conditioning regimen and then repeated on days +1, +2, and +3 post-transplant. This has been approved for use in autologous HSCT only and is used primarily with TBI-based regimens.

   d. Oral cryotherapy during and for 1 h after the administration of high-dose melphalan

   e. Artificial saliva (Caphosol®) oral rinse solutions: One ampule each of sodium phosphate and calcium chloride, combined, at least 4 times and up to 10 times daily. Patient should rinse with $\frac{1}{2}$ of solution for 1 full min and spit. Repeat with remaining $\frac{1}{2}$ of solution. Patient should refrain from oral intake for 15 min after each dose.

   f. Denture use should be minimized; dentures should be immersed in antimicrobial solution when stored with change in solution on a daily basis.

   g. Avoid use if dentures are ill fitting, abrasive to mucosa, or if there is active mucositis.

   h. Avoid hot, abrasive, sharp, or hard foods. Moisten food with sauces or gravies. Avoid hot, acidic, or carbonated liquids. Avoid artificial flavoring, especially pungent compounds such as mint and cinnamon.

   i. Maintain adequate hydration.

      i. Keep lips moist using ointment and lip moisturizers containing aloe. Avoid petroleum products.

      ii. Sucralfate (Carafate®) 1 g dissolved in solution, swish and swallow every 6 h beginning on admission has been used in some centers. Not to be used with radiation-induced OM.

17.4 MANAGEMENT OF ORAL COMPLICATIONS

1. The management of mucositis is mostly symptomatic and focused on comfort and palliation. See Table 17.2 for recommended therapies based on severity of findings.

TABLE 17.1. Stomatitis evaluation scales

Grade	WHO[a]	NCI-CTC[b]	Bearman
Grade 0	No oral abnormalities	No oral abnormalities	No oral abnormalities
Grade 1	Oral soreness ± erythema without ulcerations; able to tolerate regular diet	Erythema	Pain and/or ulceration not requiring a continuous IV narcotic drug
Grade 2	Oral soreness with erythema and ulcerations; able to tolerate solid food	Patchy ulcerations or pseudomembranes	Pain and/or ulceration requiring a continuous IV narcotic drug (morphine drip)
Grade 3	Oral soreness with erythema and ulcerations; able to tolerate liquids only	Confluent ulcerations or pseudomembranes; bleeding with minor trauma	Severe ulceration and/or mucositis requiring preventative intubation; or resulting in documented aspiration pneumonia with or without intubation
Grade 4	Oral soreness with erythema and ulcerations; unable to tolerate anything by mouth	Tissue necrosis; significant spontaneous bleeding; life-threatening consequences	Death
Grade 5	None	Death	None

[a] World Health Organization
[b] National Cancer Institute-Common Toxicity Criteria

TABLE 17.2. Management of oral complications

Symptom	Severity	Treatment
Pain	Mild	Use of bland oral rinses to maintain moisture
		Normal Saline swish and spit every 2 h
		Sodium bicarbonate solution every 2 h
		Sodium chloride rinses
		Sponge swab
		Ice chips
		Use of sialagogues
		Artificial saliva
		Sugarless hard candies or sugarless gum
		Pilocarpine 5–10 mg po TID (Salogen)
		Cevimeline 30 mg po TID
		Bethanecol 25 mg po TID
		Topical fluoride treatments
		Biotene mouthwash or toothpaste
	Moderate	Reduce oral challenges such as converting all medications to IV formula, providing IV fluid. and/or parenteral nutrition
		Topical analgesia
		Compounded mouthwashes (Maalox: Benadryl elixir: Viscous Lidocaine 1:1:1) 10–15 mL swish and spit every hour PRN
		Benzocaine gel apply topically to oral lesions QID PRN
		Doxepin 5 mg/mL 5 mL po held in the mouth for 5 min PRN
		Systemic opiates
		Scheduled opiate administration

TABLE 17.2. (*Continued*)

Symptom	Severity	Treatment
	Severe	Parenteral narcotics
		Use of narcotic patches and IV administration
		Patient-controlled analgesia
Xerostomia and hyposalivation		Use of bland oral rinses to maintain moisture
		Normal saline swish and spit PRN
		Sodium bicarbonate solution every 2 h
		Sponge swab
		Half-strength hydrogen peroxide swish and spit PRN
		Use of sialagogues
		Artificial saliva
		Sugarless hard candies or sugarless gum
		Pilocarpine 5–10 mg po TID (Salogen)
		Cevimeline 30 mg po TID
		Bethanecol 25 mg po TID
		Topical fluoride treatments
		Biotene mouthwash or toothpaste
		Caphosol swish and spit 4–10 times daily PRN

TABLE 17.2. (*Continued*)

Symptom	Severity	Treatment
Thick secretions		Use mucolytic drying agents
		Scopolamine patch TD behind ear apply every 72 h
		Dimenhydrinate 25–50 mg po every 4 h PRN
		Diphenhydramine 25–50 mg po or 12.5–25 mg IV every 6 h PRN
		Lorazepam 0.5–1 mg po/IV every 6 h PRN (gag reflex)
		Utilize suction to alleviate secretions
		Utilize blow-by humidified air
Emesis		Anti-emetics scheduled around the clock
Bleeding		Transfuse to keep platelets >20,000 for mild gingival bleeding
		Transfuse to keep platelets >50,000 for severe gingival bleeding
Airway Protection		Utilize blow-by humidified air
		Short course of IV steroids
		ENT consult for prophylactic intubation

17.5 INFECTIONS

1. Most common pathogens causing infection in patients with OM undergoing HSCT
   a. *Streptococcus viridans*
   b. Coagulase-negative Staphylococci
   c. Gram-negative bacteria
   d. Herpes simplex
   e. *Candida albicans*
   f. CMV
2. Swab and culture all oral lesions.
3. Candidal infections
   a. Topical treatments
      i. Nystatin liquid 10 mL swish and spit/swallow every 6 h
      ii. Clotrimazole (Mycelex®) troches 1 by mouth five times daily
      iii. Amphotericin mouthwash: 50 mg amphotericin B mixed in 200 mL sterile water, 5–10 mL swish and spit/swallow every 6 h.
   b. Systemic antifungals
      i. Fluconazole 400 mg po or IV daily if oral involvement
      ii. Micafungin 150 mg IV once daily if esophageal involvement and fluconazole intolerance.
4. Viral infections
   a. Systemic antivirals
      i. Acyclovir 800 mg po daily or 250 mg/m^2 IV twice daily
      ii. Valacyclovir 500 mg po twice daily
5. Bacterial
   a. Systemic antibacterials
      i. Fluroquinolone through engraftment or for periods of neutropenia >7 days
         – Ciprofloxacin 500 mg po BID
         – Levofloxacin 400 mg po daily

17.6 PRE-DENTAL PROCEDURES

The American Dental Association does not recommend prophylaxis for dental procedures for immunocompromised hosts; however, it continues to be standard practice. Common regimens:

1. Amoxicillin 2 g once prior to procedure
2. Clindamycin 600 mg once prior to procedure or QID for 10 days post procedure

3. Azithromycin 500 mg once prior to procedure or once daily for 10 days post procedure

17.7 TASTE ALTERATIONS

1. Dyegeusia (distorted taste), hypogeusia (loss of taste) or ageusia (absence of taste)
   a. Most affected are sweet and salty tastes
   b. Good oral hygiene
   c. Use artificial sialagogues
   d. Season foods
   e. Eat small portions

17.8 DISCHARGE

1. Patients may begin flossing once platelet count is >50,000.
2. Patients should be encouraged to use saline rinses for 3–6 months post-transplant as indicated.
3. Patients with GVHD should
   a. Undergo frequent dental evaluation
   b. Practice meticulous dental hygiene with use of toothbrush TID, flossing daily, dental fluoride treatments in use of sialagogues as needed.
4. Sugar-free candy or gum should be encouraged, particularly in patients with xerostomia
5. Return to routine professional dental care in 6–12 months if counts are normal. Delay elective oral procedures for 12 months.

References

Bearman, S.I., Appelbaum, F.R., Buckner, C.D., Petersen, F.B., Fisher, L.D., Clift, R.A., et al. (1988). Regimen-related toxicity in patients undergoing bone marrow transplantation. *J Clin Oncol*, 6: 1562–1568.

Bensinger, W., Schubert, M., Ang, K., Brizel, D., Brown, E., Eilers, J., et al. (2008). NCCN task force report: Prevention and management of mucositis in cancer care. *J Natl Compr Canc Netw*, 6(Suppl 1), s1–s21.

Blijlevens, N.M.A, Donnelly, J.P., DePauw, B.E. (2000). Mucosal barrier injury: Biology, pathology, clinical counterparts and consequences of intensive treatment for haematological malignancy: An overview. *Bone Marrow Transplant*, 25:1269–1278.

Boer, C.C., Correa, M.E.P., Miranda, E.C.M., de Souza, C.A. (2009). Taste disorders and oral evaluation in patients undergoing allogeneic hematopoietic stem cell transplant. *Bone Marrow Transplant*, 45:705–711.

CDC guidelines October 20, 2000/49(RR10);1–128.

Engelhard, D., Akova, M., Boeckh, M.J., Freifeld, A., Sepkowitz, K., Viscoli, C., et al. (2009). Bacterial infection prevention after hematopoietic cell transplantation. *Bone Marrow Transplant*, 44: 467–470.

Epstein, J.B, Raber-Drulacher, J.E., Wilkins, A., Chavarria, M.G., Myint, H. (2009). Advances in hematologic stem cell transplant: An update for oral health care providers. *Oral Surg Oral Med Oral Pathol Oral Radiol Endod*, 107:301–312.

Filicko, J., Lazarus, H.M., Flomenberg, N. (2003). Mucosal injury in patients undergoing hematopoietic progenitor cell transplantation: New approaches to prophylaxis and treatment. *Bone Marrow Transplant*, 31:1–10.

Keefe D.M., Schubert M.M., Elting L.S., Sonis S.T., Epstein J.B., Raber-Durlacher J.E., et al. (2007). Mucositis study section of the multinational association of supportive care in cancer and the international society for oral oncology. *Cancer*, 109:820–831.

Lockhart, P.B., Loven, B., Brennan, M.T., Fox, P.C., (2007). The evidence base for the efficacy of antibiotic prophylaxis in dental practice. *J Am Dent Assoc*, 138:458–474.

Stevens, M.M., (2005). Gastrointestinal complications of hematopoietic stem cell transplantation. In Ezzone, S. (Ed.), *Hematopoietic Stem Cell Transplantation; A Manual for Nursing Practice* (pp. 147–165). Oncology Nursing Society, Pittsburg, PA

CHAPTER 18
Gastrointestinal Complications

Eneida Nemecek

Gastrointestinal and hepatic complications are common in the hematopoietic stem cell transplant (HSCT) patient. The agents used in the conditioning regimen induce direct disruption of the intestinal barrier as well as indirect damage from cytokine release and generalized inflammatory state. These events lead to permeation of bacteria and endotoxins through the bowel wall, with subsequent organ damage and increased risk for infections. Similarly, HSCT conditioning can directly affect the hepatic parenchyma or hepatic sinusoids. The immunosuppressed state of the HSCT patient also increases the risk for opportunistic infections of the gastrointestinal tract and liver.

This chapter includes information describing potential gastrointestinal and hepatic complications that may arise in the HSCT patient and provides guidelines for their management.

18.1 UPPER GASTROINTESTINAL
1. Anorexia
   a. Etiology and pathogenesis
      Usual onset during conditioning and first week post-transplant; may last longer in patients with mucositis, infection, or GvHD. May result from
      i. Direct emetogenic effect from conditioning therapy
      ii. Delayed gastric emptying
      iii. Circulating inflammatory cytokines directly affecting appetite centers
      iv. Mucositis-related pain and dysphagia, graft-versus-host disease

R.T. Maziarz, S. Slater (eds.), *Blood and Marrow Transplant Handbook*, DOI 10.1007/978-1-4419-7506-5_18, © Springer Science+Business Media, LLC 2011

   v. Infection

   vi. Medications

  b. Diagnosis

   Most cases are identified by clinical presentation and do not require additional workup. Endoscopic evaluation (i.e., esophagogastroduodenoscopy) with biopsies to identify potential underlying causes is recommended for cases of protracted or prolonged nausea, vomiting, or anorexia after mucositis has resolved.

  c. Treatment

   i. Conditioning regimens for HSCT are in general considered as highly emetogenic therapy. Antiemetic prophylaxis during conditioning therapy (see Chapter 5) should aim at minimizing nausea and vomiting and preserving enteral nutrition for as long as possible. Management of nausea and vomiting are discussed in Chapter 6.

   ii. Daily calorie count to determine whether (a) adequate nutritional goals are achieved and (b) to identify if there may be need for enteral or parenteral supplementation (see Chapter 7).

   iii. The efficacy of appetite stimulants in the post-transplant setting has not been determined and is generally not recommended. However, if anorexia becomes chronic, one could consider a trial of megestrol (Megace®) acetate oral solution 800 mg/day, dronabinol (Marinol®) 2.5 to 5 mg po before lunch and dinner or mirtazipine (Remeron®) 7.5–45 mg po qhs. The safety and efficacy of these agents in children have not been established, although empiric use has been reported. Consultation with a pediatric pharmacist prior to their use is recommended.

2. Esophagitis/gastritis

  a. Etiology and pathogenesis

   Usually presents during conditioning and period of mucositis, but may last longer in patients with GVHD. Potential etiologies include

   i Mucositis

   ii. Medications

   iii. Poor oral intake

   iv. Altered gastric pH

   v. "True" peptic ulcer disease

  b. Diagnosis

   Diagnosis is clinical. Symptoms are usually heartburn and/or epigastric pain.

c. Treatment
  i. First-line of therapy is elevation of the head of bed and antacids (calcium carbonate, magnesium or aluminum hydroxide).
  ii. H_2-blockers (ranitidine, cimetidine) should be avoided in the first 100 days post-transplant due to their myelosuppressive potential.
  iii. Proton-pump inhibitors may be of utility in patients with gastritis symptoms. However, their use should be reserved for patients failing first-line treatment and limited to 7–10 days, as prolonged use may inhibit the natural antimicrobial barrier and increase the risk for infection.
    – Lansoprazole (Prevacid®) 30–60 mg po daily to BID
    – Omeprazole (Prilosec®) 20–40 mg po daily to BID
    – Pantoprazole (Protonix®) 40–80 mg po daily
  iv. Gastric acid blockade therapy can impact the absorption of coincident oral azole antifungal prophylaxis.

18.2 LOWER GASTROINTESTINAL

1. Diarrhea
  a. Etiology and pathogenesis
  Can present anytime during conditioning or post-transplant. The time of onset is usually a hint for potential etiologies. Potential etiologies include
    i. Direct side effect from conditioning and other medications
    ii. Mucositis and intestinal epithelial sloughing
    iii. Infection
    iv. GvHD
    v. Pancreatic insufficiency
    vi. Brush border disaccharidase deficiency
    vii. Malabsorption
    viii. Intestinal thrombotic microangiopathy
    ix. Mycophenolate mofetil (Cellcept®) is a very common inciting agent (through direct mucosal toxicity) and may be very difficult to distinguish from GvHD.
  b. Diagnosis
  Rule out infection with stool cultures for enteric pathogens. For patients in which diarrhea does not improve after resolution of oral mucositis, consideration for rectosigmoidoscopy to perform visual inspection and obtain tissue biopsies is recommended.

   c. Treatment
      i. Identify and treat the underlying cause.
      ii. Supportive care should focus on hydration and prevention/treatment of electrolyte imbalances.
      iii. Bowel rest/restricted diet (low roughage, low residue; low or no lactose).
      iv. Calculate and replace enteral volume losses with isotonic fluid.
      v. Monitor and replace protein losses (albumin, gammaglobulin).
      vi. Vitamin K depletion in chronic diarrhea is common. If the prothrombin time is elevated, vitamin K should be replaced. The dose is 2.5–25 mg IV or SQ (max 10 mg for children); if prothrombin time is not satisfactory within 6–8 h, the dose may be repeated.
      vii. Oral loperamide (Imodium® 2–4 mg every 6 h) or intravenous octreotide may be effective to treat or relieve diarrhea associated with conditioning regimen and GvHD. The recommended octreotide (Sandostatin®) regimen varies. A fixed dose of 500 mcg every 8 h for 7 days or 50 mcg (2 mcg/kg) intravenously 3 times per day escalated to continuous infusion at 15 mcg/h (1 mcg/kg/h) have been reported to have some success in control of diarrhea in the transplant setting.
      viii. Anti-diarrheal agents should not be used in patients with infectious diarrhea. Negative stool studies (bacterial, viral, *Clostridium difficile* toxin assay) should be ascertained prior to the addition of antimotility agents.
2. Gastrointestinal bleeding
   a. Etiology and pathogenesis
   Most cases have diffuse areas of bleeding as opposed to a localized site. Causes of GI bleeding include:
      i. Thrombocytopenia
      ii. Esophageal trauma (from retching)
      iii. Esophagitis
      iv. Colitis
      v. Anal fissures or hemorrhoids
      vi. Viral infections
      vii. GVHD
   b. Diagnosis
   Diagnosis is clinical. An esophagogastroduodenoscopy with rectosigmoidoscopy/colonoscopy may aid in

identifying the cause of bleeding and to deliver local bleeding control.

c. Treatment

If possible, treatment of the underlying cause should be initiated. Symptom control can be achieved with:

 i. Platelet support (keeping platelets at least over 50,000/mm^3)

 ii. PRBC transfusion to maintain hematocrit >28%

 iii. Octreotide IV may provide short-term control.

 iv. Local bleeding control with endoscopic cautery or embolization (if localized disease)

 v. If large-volume acute blood loss, consider desmopressin (DDAVP) or aminocaproic acid (Amicar®), providing the patient has no evidence of hematuria. The use of recombinant factor VII to control bleeding in the transplant setting has not been studied and its routine use is not recommended.

 vi. Consider radiologic assessment with angiography or a red cell nuclear scan to identify areas of active bleeding.

18.3 HEPATOBILIARY DISEASES

1. Sinusoidal obstruction syndrome or venoocclusive disease of the liver (SOS/VOD)

 a. Epidemiology

 Incidence is reported at approximately 5–10%. Severe SOS/VOD frequently leads to multi-organ failure and is associated with day-100 mortality of over 90%.

 b. Etiology and pathogenesis

 Usually presents during the first weeks following conditioning, prior to engraftment, and results from direct injury to sinusoidal endothelial cells and hepatocytes. Pre-transplant risk factors include:

 i. Older age (or younger age for children)

 ii. Poor performance status

 iii. Female gender

 iv. Advanced malignancy or patients with inherited disorders of metabolism

 v. Reduced pulmonary diffusion capacity (DLCO)

 vi. Prior hepatic disease (elevated bilirubin or AST, preexisting cirrhosis)

 vii. Prior abdominal radiation

    viii. Use of gemtuzumab ozogamicin (Mylotarg®) within 3 months of conditioning

c. Transplant risk factors include:
    i. Myeloablative conditioning
    ii. Second transplant
    iii. Use of high-dose alkylating chemotherapy or TBI
    iv. Use of methotrexate for GvHD prophylaxis.

d. Diagnosis
    i. Clinical picture includes:
      – Total bilirubin >2 mg/dL,
      – Weight gain >5% from baseline.
      – Right upper quadrant tenderness (tender hepatomegaly) ± ascites.
    ii. Abdominal ultrasound with liver Doppler usually shows hepatomegaly, ascites, and, in more advanced cases, reversal of portal flow.
    iii. Liver biopsy is not necessary for diagnosis. If needed to rule out other causes, a transvenous liver biopsy with measurement of hepatic venous pressure gradient should be obtained. More invasive procedures (percutaneous or open biopsy) carry higher risk due to high pressures and potential coagulopathy associated with hepatic synthetic dysfunction.
    vi. Differential diagnoses include: sepsis-related cholestasis, other cholestatic liver disease, and graft-versus-host disease.

e. Treatment
    i. Prevention of SOS is the best intervention by recognizing patients who are at risk for this toxicity and, when possible, avoiding exposure to known risk factors (i.e., selection of transplant conditioning regimen).
    ii. Ursodeoxycholic acid (Ursodiol®) 300 mg po BID (6 mg/kg/dose for children) from start of conditioning until approximately 1 week after engraftment has been shown in small randomized studies of prophylaxis to provide benefit in decreasing the severity of SOS/VOD.
    iii. Prompt treatment is crucial, as the severe form of this disease results in very high rates of mortality (70–80%).
    iv. Supportive care is the standard treatment, including

- Maintaining careful fluid (water and sodium) balance.
- Providing aggressive diuresis.
- Discontinuing/avoiding agents that may exacerbate hepatotoxicity, when possible.
- Preserving renal blood flow (renal dose dopamine 2–5 mcg/kg/min), if needed.
  v. Defibrotide is a potent antithrombotic and profibrinolytic agent. A historical-controlled phase 3 study demonstrated a survival advantage for patients with severe SOS who receive this drug early in the course of their disease. This agent is not commercially available in the United States yet, but can be procured under compassionate, emergency use.
2. Acute hepatitis (also see Chapter 14)
   a. Etiology and pathogenesis
   Can present anytime during conditioning or post-transplant. The time of onset is usually a hint for potential etiologies, which includes:
   i. Infection/sepsis
   ii. Acute biliary obstruction
   iii. Drug-induced toxicity
   iv. GvHD
   b. Diagnosis
   i. Sudden elevation of serum transaminases (AST, ALT)
   ii. Blood tests for viral DNA (herpes viruses, adenovirus, hepatitis B)
   iii. Imaging (CT or ultrasound) may be used to identify fungal abscesses in the case of infection.
   iv. Liver biopsy may aid in identifying a cause.
   c. Treatment
   Supportive care, removal of inciting agents (if drug-related, when possible), treatment of infection.
   i. A prolonged course of antibiotics or antifungals may be needed for bacterial or fungal infections.
   ii. Acute viral hepatitis may lead to fulminant hepatic failure if not treated promptly. Possible viruses include herpes, varicella, cytomegalovirus, and human-herpes viruses (HHV-6 and HHV-8). If the patient is not on acyclovir prophylaxis, initiation of empiric treatment is recommended.
   iii. Hepatitis B can also present with fulminant hepatic failure. Patients with previous history of hepatitis B or exposed to a donor with previous history of hepatitis

B are at higher risk. Antiviral therapy should be initiated promptly (lamivudine, tenofovir, or similar). The initiation and further dosing for these agents should be determined with the assistance of the Gastroenterologist/Hepatologist).

3. Gall bladder disease and pancreatitis
   a. Etiology and pathogenesis
      Biliary sludging is very common in transplant patients and is usually asymptomatic, but may also cause acute acalculous cholecystitis, pancreatitis, or cholangitis. Sludging may result from:
      i. Chemotherapy
      ii. Parenteral alimentation with prolonged absence of oral intake
      iii. Antibiotics
      iv. Hyperlipidemia
      v. GvHD.
   b. Diagnosis
      Abdominal ultrasound may reveal gall bladder disease (thickening of gallbladder wall, stones, etc.). Radionuclide bile excretion study (HIDA scan) may reveal gall bladder obstruction.
   c. Treatment
      i. Bowel rest
      ii. Removal of parenteral alimentation, if inciting agent
      iii. Cholecystectomy is infrequently needed
      iv. Endoscopic retrograde cholangiopancreatography (ERCP) is only needed in the case of obstructive cholangitis

References

Barker, C., Anderson, R., Sauve, R., Butzner, J. (2005). GI complications in pediatric patients post-BMT. *Bone Marrow Transplant*, 36(1): 51–58.

Bresters, D., Van Gils, I., Dekker, F., Lankester, A., Bredius, R., Schweizer, J. (2008). Abnormal liver enzymes 2 years after haematopoietic stem cell transplantation in children: Prevalence and risk factors. *Bone Marrow Transplant*, 41(1):27–31.

Cox, G., Matsui, S., Lo, R., Hinds, M., Bowden, R., Hackman, R., et al. (1994). Etiology and outcome of diarrhea after marrow transplantation; a prospective study. *Gastroenterology*, 107(5):1398–1407.

Crouch, M., Restino, M., Cruz, J., Perry, J., Hurd, D. (1996). Octreotide acetate in refractory bone marrow transplant-associated diarrhea. *Ann Pharmacothera*, 30(4):331–336.

Firpi, R., Nelson, D. (2006). Viral hepatitis: Manifestations and management strategy. *Hematology Am Soc Hematol Educ Program*, 375–380.

Geller, R., Gilmore, C., Dix, S., Lin, L., Topping, D., Davidson, T., et al. (1995). Randomized trial of loperimide versus dose escalation of octreotide acetate for chemotherapy-induced diarrhea in bone marrow transplant and leukemia patients. *Am J Hematol*, 50(3):167–172.

Ho, V., Revta, C., Richardson, P. (2008). Hepatic veno-occlusive disease after hematopoietic stem cell transplantation: Update on defibrotide and other current investigational therapies. Bone Marrow Transplant, 41(3):229–237.

Ippoliti, C., Champlin, R., Bugazia, N., Przepiorka, D., Neumann, J., Giralt, S., et al. (1997). Use of octreotide in the symptomatic management of diarrhea induced by graft-versus-host disease in patients with hematologic malignancies. *J Clin Oncol*, 5(11): 3350–3354.

Johansson, J., Abrahamsson, H., Ekman, T. (2003). Gastric emptying after autologous hematopoietic stem cell transplantation: A prospective trial. *Bone Marrow Transplant*, 32(8):815–819.

Ko, C., Gooley, T., Schoch, H., Myerson, D., Hackman, R., Shulman, H., et al. (1997). Acute pancreatitis in marrow transplant patients: Prevalence at autopsy and risk factor analysis. *Bone Marrow Transplant*, 20(12):1081–1086.

Malone, F., Leisenring, W., Storer, B. L., Stern, J., Bouvier, M., Martin, P., et al. (2007). Prolonged anorexia and elevated plasma cytokine levels following myeloablative allogeneic hematopoietic cell transplant. *Bone Marrow Transplant*, 40(8):765–772.

Murray, S., Pindoria, S. (2009, January 21). *Nurtrition support for bone marrow transplant patients*. Retrieved from mrw.interscience.wiley.com: CD002920.

Sakai, M., Strasser, S., Shulman, H., McDonald, S., Schoch, H., McDonald, G. (2009). Severe hepatocellular injury after hematopoietic stem cell transplant: Incidence, etiology and outcome. *Bone Marrow Transplant*, 44(7):441–447.

Schulenburg, A., Turetschedk, K., Wrba, F., Vogelsang, H., Greinix, H., Keil, F., et al. (2004). Early and late gastrointestinal complications after myeloablative and nonmyeloablative allogeneic stem cell transplantation. *Ann Hematol*, 83(2):101–106.

Schwartz, J., Wolford, J., Thornquist, M., Hockenbery, D., Murakami, C., Drennan, F., et al. (2001). Severe gastrointestinal bleeding after hematopoietic stem cell transplantation, 1987–1997: Incidence, causes, and outcome. *Am J Gastroenterol*, 96(2):385–393.

Teefey, S., Hollister, M., Lee, S., Jacobson, A., Higano, C., Bianco, J., et al. (1994). Gallbladder sludge formation after bone marrow transplant: Sonographic observations. *Abdom Imaging*, 19(1): 57–60.

CHAPTER 19
Pulmonary Complications

Tarek Eid and Alan F. Barker

After hematopoietic stem cell transplant (HSCT), up to 60% of patients develop pulmonary complications. In spite of antibacterial, antiviral, and antifungal prophylaxis, reduced host defenses render the HSCT patient vulnerable to pulmonary and other infections in the early weeks and even months post-transplantation. This chapter will suggest an integrative approach followed by a description of the most common pulmonary syndromes seen in HSCT patients, including diffuse alveolar hemorrhage (DAH), idiopathic pneumonia syndrome (IPS), bronchiolitis obliterans syndrome (BO or BOS), and cryptogenic organizing pneumonia (COP).

Investigating new pulmonary complaints is challenging. All patients should undergo an extensive workup of new pulmonary findings, including dyspnea, cough, fever, and hypoxia. In the first 4–6 weeks post-transplant, neutropenic patients can develop bacterial pneumonia. Pathogens include Gram-negative rods (*Pseudomonas* or *Klebsiella*), *Staphylococcus aureus*, and *Nocardia*. While chest x-rays could show typical lobar or multilobar opacities, CT scan of the chest (noncontrast CT scans are adequate for workup of infectious processes) may yield additional characteristic findings (nodules, ground glass opacities, etc.). Fungal pneumonias, primarily *Aspergillus*, can also develop in this early period. There is a very strong association between invasive *Aspergillus* pneumonia and neutropenia lasting more than 10 days. Viral pneumonia may develop as well in this patient population; however, it tends to occur later. CMV is the most common viral pathogen, but with monitoring and preemptive therapy, the incidence has declined. Other

R.T. Maziarz, S. Slater (eds.), *Blood and Marrow Transplant Handbook*, DOI 10.1007/978-1-4419-7506-5_19, © Springer Science+Business Media, LLC 2011

viruses that have emerged as pathogens include RSV, influenza, and parainfluenza (see Chapter 14).

19.1 BRONCHOSCOPY

Bronchoalveolar lavage (BAL) via bronchoscopy should be pursued once pneumonia is considered. Pre-procedure stabilization with supplemental oxygen is key. Depressed mental status may increase the risk of the procedure. The presence of severe hypoxia and depressed mental status may require endotracheal intubation to safely perform the procedure. Unless there is active bleeding, correction of coagulopathy is not required, and there is no absolute platelet level required for safety with BAL alone. If transbronchial biopsy will be attempted, a pre-procedure platelet count of $\geq 30,000/mm^3$ and INR of <1.5 is recommended. Conscious sedation with fentanyl and/or midazolam is often used for comfort and amnesia. Complications of bronchoscopy include worsening hypoxemia, airway hemorrhage, and respiratory failure. The risks with transbronchial biopsy are much higher including pneumothorax, respiratory failure, and difficult to control airway bleeding.

Appropriately stained BAL smears may suggest a pathogen in a matter of hours while cytology, culture, and genetic results are pending. BAL fluid should routinely be sent for:

1. Cytology including stains for organisms (fungi, PCP); stain for hemosiderin laden macrophages
2. Bacterial cultures (including *Nocardia*) and sensitivity
3. Fungal smear and culture
4. Mycobacterium smear and culture
5. Cell count and differential
6. Galactomannan antigen
7. PCR for respiratory viral panels
8. PCR for legionella
9. DFA staining for PCP

19.2 DIFFUSE ALVEOLAR HEMORRHAGE (DAH)

DAH is a subset of pulmonary hemorrhage that can develop in up to 5% of all post hematopoietic stem cell transplants with mortality rates ranging between 50 and 80% based on the two largest case series. About 87% of the cases develop in the first 3 weeks post-HSCT.

1. Risk factors
   a. Advanced age
   b. Grade 3–4 acute graft-versus-host disease (GvHD)
   c. Allogeneic transplant
   d. Pre-transplant conventional myeloablative regimen
   e. Thrombocytopenia
   f. Renal insufficiency
   g. Coagulopathy
2. Clinical findings
   a. Shortness of breath
   b. Cough
   c. Rarely hemoptysis
   d. Fever
   e. Tachypnea
   f. Acrocyanosis
   g. Crackles heard on lung auscultation
3. Diagnostic tests
   a. Chest x-ray often shows bilateral diffuse alveolar opacities, which could be confirmed by CT scan imaging (Fig. 19.1) as ground glass opacities. These findings are not specific as can be seen in many other conditions.
   b. Pulmonary function testing shows increased DLCO; however, often these patients cannot participate in such testing.
   c. Bronchoscopy with bronchoalveolar lavage is the confirmatory diagnostic method. Bronchoalveolar lavage shows progressive bloody return. Cytology with Prussian blue staining should show >20% hemosiderin laden macrophages. This test is limited if alveolar hemorrhage happened less than 48–72 hours before the procedure, as macrophages may not take up enough RBCs.
4. Pathogenesis of DAH
   There is no clear etiology for DAH post-HSCT. The development of DAH around the engraftment period suggests an inflammatory cascade involving the alveoli. Pre-transplant conditioning regimens (including total body irradiation) may initiate the inflammatory process.
5. Management
   Transferring such patients to the medical intensive care unit is recommended, given that respiratory failure can develop rapidly. Some patients require high-flow oxygen and subsequent mechanical ventilation for acute respiratory distress

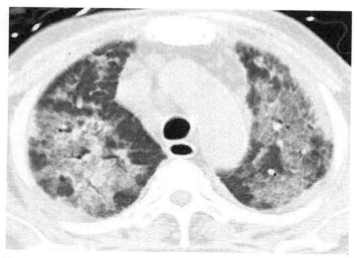

FIG. 19.1. Diffuse grand ground opacities in diffuse alveolar hemorrhage, confirmed by BAL

syndrome (ARDS). Supportive management and high-dose systemic steroids are the key parts of DAH treatment.

a. Mechanical ventilation should be tailored to each individual, reflecting the ARDS mechanical ventilation protocol/low tidal volume for acute lung injury.

b. Immunosuppressive therapy with high-dose corticosteroids is the mainstay of therapy based on case reports and retrospective series. Doses of up to 1 g of methylprednisone divided into 2–4 doses should be given daily for 3–5 days, followed by a slow taper over 1–3 months. Alternate dosing schedules have been suggested, beginning at 2 mg/kg daily in divided doses, tapering over a 2-month period.

c. Correction of underlying coagulopathy by maintaining platelet count above $50,000/mm^3$ and INR <2.

d. Examine for concomitant infectious pathogen using bronchoalveolar lavage.

e. Recombinant factor VIIa has been tried with no change in patient's outcome.

f. Aminocaproic acid has been used less frequently and with limited supporting data.

19.3 IDIOPATHIC PNEUMONIA SYNDROME (IPS)

IPS is severe lung injury that develops after allogeneic hematopoietic stem cell transplant with no evidence of infectious process. The incidence ranges between 2 and 35%, with mortality rates ranging from 60 to 80%. If mechanical ventilation becomes necessary, mortality approaches 95%. The time course for developing IPS is post-transplant in the first 2 months; however, delayed onset has been reported. See Table 19.1 for different acronyms of interstitial lung diseases.

TABLE 19.1   Selected acronyms of Interstitial lung disease

Acronym	Interstitial lung disease
UIP/IPF	Usual interstitial pneumonitis/idiopathic pulmonary fibrosis
HSP	Hypersensitivity pneumonitis (often due to an aeroallergen such as thermophilic fungi)
NSIP	Nonspecific interstitial pneumonitis
IPS	Idiopathic pneumonia syndrome
BOS	Bronchiolitis obliterans syndrome
BOOP/COP	Bronchiolitis obliterans organizing pneumonia/cryptogeneic organizing pneumonia
AIP	Acute interstitial pneumonia

1. Risk factors
   a. Grade 3–4 acute graft-versus-host disease (GvHD)
   b. Donor CMV positivity
   c. Conditioning regimens containing total body irradiation
   d. Older age
   e. Certain malignancies (acute leukemia, myelodysplastic syndrome)
   f. Drug toxicity has been implicated; however, there is no method to discriminate between drug-induced lung damage and IPS.
2. Clinical findings
   Findings are indistinguishable from pneumonia, which include fever, cough usually productive or scant of no phlegm, shortness of breath, and hypoxia.
3. Diagnostic tests
   The criteria for diagnosis of IPS proposed by the National Heart Lung and Blood Institute in 1993 include:
   a. Radiologic imaging evidence of multlilobar diffuse alveolar infiltrates

    b. Hypoxia or elevated alveolar-arterial gradient

    c. Negative bronchoalveolar lavage for blood and cultures for bacteria, fungi, and viruses

    d. Negative infectious studies from the blood specifically for CMV

    e. Negative transbronchial biopsy for infectious causes performed 2–14 days after the initial negative BAL

    All patients with suspected IPS should undergo chest imaging and bronchoscopy with BAL to rule out infection. Occasionally, chest imaging does not show obvious infiltrates, and CT scan of the chest is warranted.

4. Pathogenesis of IPS

    Evaluation of BAL fluid from IPS patients shows elevated inflammatory cytokine markers compared to negative or healthy controls.

5. Management

    a. Corticosteroids should be started early in the disease course. Historically, patients who developed IPS around engraftment responded better to steroids. A reasonable starting dose is 2 mg/kg daily of prednisolone for the first week, followed by a slow taper over the course of 2–3 months.

    b. PCP and fungal prophylaxis are recommended.

    c. Etanercept (Enbrel®) 25 mg SQ twice weekly for 8 weeks has been used in conjunction with corticosteroids with some success in small case series.

19.4 BRONCHIOLITIS OBLITERANS SYNDROME (BOS)

The most common late complication following allogeneic HSCT is BOS. Eighty percent of the cases occur 6–12 months post-transplant. Incidence varies considerably, but may be as high as 40%. BOS is rarely reported after autologous HSCT or umbilical cord blood stem cell transplant. Almost all patients have manifestations of GvHD. Most authors consider BOS as GvHD of the lung. It is also important to recognize BOS as a separate clinical entity from bronchiolitis obliterans with organizing pneumonia, also known as cryptogenic organizing pneumonia (BOOP or COP). See Table 19.1.

1. Risk factors reported by the CIBMTR include:

    a. Blood-derived stem cells

    b. Busulfan-based conditioning regimen

    c. Interval from diagnosis of leukemia to transplantation of less than 14 months

    d. Female donor to male recipient

    e. Prior interstitial pneumonitis

    f. An episode of grade 3–4 acute GvHD

    Additional risk factors include

    g. Prior allogeneic HSCT

    h. Older age

    i. Prior airflow obstruction

    j. Previous respiratory viral infection (CMV)

    k. IgG level <400 results in a two- to threefold risk of developing BOS

2. Definition

The NIH diagnosis and staging working group prepared a consensus definition for BOS, so further studies can utilize the same inclusion criteria:

    a. Absence of active infection

    b. Decreased FEV1 (<75% of predicted normal)

    c. Evidence of airway obstruction with a ratio of FEV1/FVC <0.7

    d. Elevated residual volume (>120% of predicted normal)

    e. Expiratory chest CT that reveals air trapping or bronchiectasis

    f. Lung biopsy typically shows cicatricial bronchial obliterans (i.e., obliteration of airways by dense fibrous scar tissues)

3. Clinical findings

Insidious course manifested by nonproductive cough, wheezing, and dyspnea. Early in BOS respiratory physical exam might be normal; however, later stages are manifested by wheezing, prolonged expiratory phase, and inspiratory crackles.

4. Diagnostic tests

    a. Chest imaging should be carried out in all patients undergoing workup for BOS. Chest x-rays could be normal early in BOS. As the disease progresses, hyperinflation might be present.

    b. More sensitive is the high-resolution CT (HRCT) (Figs. 19.2, 19.3) of the chest including inspiratory and expiratory phases that show air trapping or "mosaic lung appearance," which indicates regional airflow obstruction during the expiratory phase.

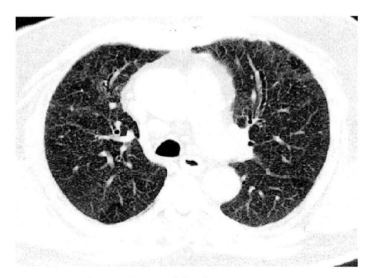

FIG. 19.2. Inspiratory CT scan of the chest

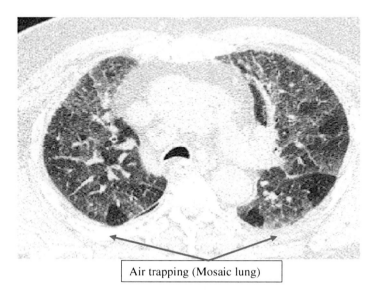

Air trapping (Mosaic lung)

FIG. 19.3. Expiratory phase CT scan chest in a patient with BOS

   c. Pulmonary function testing is obtained on patient's pre-transplant evaluation as baseline. The definition of airflow obstruction include FEV1 <75%, FEV1/FVC < 0.70, or a decline in FEV1 >20% in 1 year. Also noted is air trapping or increased residual volume (RV) and residual volume to total lung capacity (RV:TLC) ratio. DLCO is not expected to be reduced, but is often low pre-transplant and/or after induction chemotherapy.

   d. Bronchoscopy is not routinely performed during the workup of BOS, unless imaging is suspicious for an infectious process. Transbronchial biopsy is often nondiagnostic as the disease process is patchy, and if needed surgical lung biopsy has higher chance of demonstrating constrictive bronchioloitis. With the introduction of HRCT, surgical lung biopsy is not required to confirm a diagnosis of BOS.

5. Pathogenesis of BOS

   BOS may be a manifestation of primarily chronic GvHD, with the etiology related to recognition of disparate antigens present in the context of HLA class I and class II. Histopathology and clinic course of BOS are similar in respiratory and HSCT patients. It begins with fibroproliferative disease of the small airways, which results in inflammation, epithelial metaplasia, and denudification. Submucosal/mucosal fibrosis then develops, resulting in obliteration of the airways.

6. Management

   Management of BOS mainly involves intensifying immunosuppressive therapy and supportive care. There have not been any specific recommendations associated with treatment of BOS. The management of BOS mimics that of chronic GVHD, starting with:

   a. Response to bronchodilators is often minimal, but nevertheless should be considered because of the presence of airflow obstruction.

   b. Corticosteroids 1–1.5 mg/kg prednisone per day for 2–6 weeks, then tapered over 6–12 months if there is a response. This regimen is based on case series and expert opinions.

   c. Other immunosuppressive medications may be effective as steroid-sparing agents including calcineurin inhibitors. There have been no randomized control studies.

d. Macrolides have been used in BOS that develops post lung transplant. Small case series have reported improvement in FEV1 in BOS post-HSCT. Azithromycin 250 mg three times each week is a suggested regimen.

e. Leukotrienes have been reported to be elevated in BAL fluid of patients with BOS. Trials of montelukast, a leukotriene inhibitor, are underway.

f. Patients should be assessed for oxygen needs using 6-min walk test and/or nocturnal O2 monitor study.

g. Echocardiogram can screen for pulmonary hypertension and left ventricular dysfunction, both accompanied by dyspnea.

The management of BOS requires a multispecialty approach (bone marrow, pulmonary, radiology specialists). Prognosis of progressive BOS (>10% FEV1 decline per year) is poor. Two year overall survival was 45% in 2003, with a 5-year survival rate of only 13%. The majority of patients die of respiratory failure triggered by infection. Attention to dyspnea and liberal use of pulmonary function testing may allow earlier identification and treatment of BOS before permanent (fibrotic) airway changes, respiratory insufficiency, and pneumonia occur.

19.5 CRYPTOGENIC ORGANIZING PNEUMONIA (COP)

COP or bronchiolitis obliterans with organizing pneumonia (BOOP) is a disease process of unknown etiology that differs from BOS. One case series of open lung biopsies done in patients who underwent HSCT found that COP was the most common inflammatory pathology (9/17 diagnoses = 52%). One retrospective study identified the cause of COP in 50% of the cases and were listed as: radiation, chemotherapy, connective tissue disease, inhalational drugs (cocaine), Amiodarone, and inflammatory bowel disease.

1. Clinical findings
   The presentation of COP is similar to many respiratory disorders; most commonly dyspnea is accompanied by nonproductive cough, with fever also present in about 45% of patients. Physical exam is primarily notable for crackles.

2. Diagnostic tests
   a. Chest x-ray

     b. Pulmonary function testing, shows a mixed pattern of obstruction, restriction, or occasionally normal physiology

     c. CT scan of the chest is typically required to demonstrate areas of bilateral organizing pneumonia and consolidation in subpleural or peribronchial distribution associated with areas of ground glass opacities. Migratory opacities on CT scan chest have been described in 25% of patients with COP.

     d. Lung biopsy is occasionally needed. Typical pathology shows intraluminal plugs of alveolar ducts associated with surrounding chronic inflammation and organizing pneumonia.

3. Management

     a. Prognosis of COP or BOOP is favorable

     b. Bronchoscopy with BAL is often required to rule out infectious processes

     c. Corticosteriods have been used and clinical responses have been reported in 80% of cases

References

Bekele, A., Ayalew, T., Mark, R., Michael, J., Mark, E., Steve, G. (2002). Diffuse alveolar hemorrhage in hematopoietic stem cell transplant recipients. *Am J Respir Crit Care Med*, 166:641–645.

Clark, J., Hansen, J., Hertz, M., Parkman, R., Jensen, L., Peavy, H. (1993). NHLBI workshop summary. Idiopathic pneumonia syndrome after bone marrow transplantation. *Am Rev Resp Diseases*, 147:1601–1606.

Fukuda, T., Hackman, R. G., Sandmaier, B., Boeckh, M., Maris, M., Maloney, D., et al. (2003). Risks and outcomes of idiopathic pneumonia syndrome after nonmyeloablative and conventional conditioning regimens for allogeneic hematopoietic stem cell transplanation. *Blood*, 102:2777–2785.

Gupta, S., Jain, A., Warneke, C., Gupta, A., Shannon, V., Morice, R., et al. (2007). Outcome of alveolar hemorrhage in hematopoietic stem cell transplant recipients. *Bone Marrow Transplant*, 40:71–78.

Kotloff, R., Ahya, V., Crawford, S. (2004). Pulmonary complications of solid organ and stem cell transplantation. *Am J Resp Crit Care Med*, 170:22–48.

Silva, C, Muller, N. (2009). Idiopathic interstitial pneumonias. *J Thorac Imaging*, 24:260–273.

Soubani, A., Uberti, J. (2007). Bronchiolitis obliterans following hematopoietic stem cell transplantation. *Eur Respir J*, 29: 1007–1019.

Vasu, ST., Cavalazzi, R., Hirani, A., Kane, K, (2009) Clinical and radiologic distinctions between secondary bronchiolitis obliterans organizing pneumonia and cryptogenic organizing pneumonia. *Resp Care*, 1028–1032.

Williams, K., Chien, J. G., Pavletic, S. (2009). Bronchiolitis obliterans after allogenetic hematopoietic stem cell transplantation. *JAMA*, 302:306–314.

CHAPTER 20
Cardiovascular Complications

Christopher Greenman

Hematopoietic stem cell transplant (HSCT) patients face an array of proximate and remote cardiovascular events, including congestive heart failure (CHF), coronary vascular disease (CAD), pericardial disease, and arrhythmias. Toxicities may be classified temporally, appearing in acute (<2 weeks), early (2 weeks–3 months), or late (>3 months) periods following HSCT. These patients appear to be at increased risk for both subclinical and overt cardiovascular toxicities. Studies have been inconsistent in estimating the amount of clinically relevant risk, with reports ranging from no increased risk to greater than 40%. Variability in the incidence of cardiac events reported in the literature results from small patient populations, lack of matched controls, indirect measures of cardiac dysfunction, and improvements in cardiac disease management over time.

Potential causes of HSCT-associated cardiovascular disease include pre-transplant conditioning treatments such as high-dose (HD) cyclophosphamide; allogeneic versus autologous transplant status; critical illness related to HSCT status; infusion of cryopreserved marrow; and preexisting cardiovascular disease. The relative contribution that each of these factors has on total cardiac disease burden in this patient population has not been well defined.

20.1 PRE-TRANSPLANT CARDIAC EVALUATION
1. Most centers recommend screening baseline cardiac status prior to HSCT, including resting electrocardiograms (ECG) exercise ECG, chest X-ray, and echocardiogram, resting or

R.T. Maziarz, S. Slater (eds.), *Blood and Marrow Transplant Handbook*, DOI 10.1007/978-1-4419-7506-5_20, © Springer Science+Business Media, LLC 2011

with exercise. Up to 20% of HSCT candidates have evidence of subclinical cardiovascular disease based on radionuclide ventriculography.

2. Factors that have been associated with a significant incidence of cardiac toxicities following HSCT include decreased baseline ejection fraction (<40%) and prolonged QTc (>500 ms).

3. Baseline cardiac dysfunction does not reliably predict the poorest outcomes following HSCT and should not necessarily be used as an absolute contraindication to proceeding with a potentially life-saving transplant.

20.2 INCIDENCE AND TYPES OF ACUTE TOXICITY

1. Greater than 80% of fatal cardiac events occurring within the first 100 days of transplant occur in the first 2 weeks.

2. Roughly half of acute cardiac fatalities are due to CHF, which is most closely associated with high-dose cyclophosphamide. Evidence of this toxicity has been found on postmortem examinations of heart tissue. Incidence of CHF in patients receiving HD cyclophosphamide is independent of cumulative drug exposure, and multifractionated scheduling may be protective. Following infusion of HD cyclophosphamide, a drop in QRS voltage by 50% is common and usually transient. Dosing by ideal body weight has been adopted as standard to decrease the cardiotoxicity. Pretransplant anthracycline exposure is also associated with the development of acute CHF.

3. Other acute cardiac toxicities include pericardial effusion with tamponade, cardiac arrest, acute myocardial infarction, and atrial fibrillation with hemodynamic compromise.

4. Supraventricular tachyarrhythmias are reported as occurring in as many as 4% of patients in the first week following transplantation. Since tachyarrhythmias causing hemodynamic compromise are most often reported, the incidence of all tachyarrhythmias is likely much higher.

5. Tachyarrhythmias may be mediated by intrinsic heart damage, systemic circulating factors related to critical illness, or intravascular volume shifts.

20.3 BASIC PRESENTATION, WORKUP, AND TREATMENT OF COMMON ACUTE CARDIAC TOXICITIES

1. Monitoring of HSCT patients undergoing conventional myeloablative conditioning occurs initially in the hospital

followed by frequent outpatient visits, allowing for the detection of cardiovascular disease.

2. CHF occurs when the heart cannot adequately pump blood forward through the vasculature to meet the body's metabolic demands or when this can only occur with abnormally high ventricular filling pressures.

   a. CHF may present with fatigue, weight gain, dyspnea (may be worse when laying supine and often awaking patients at night), right upper quadrant pain (from congestive hepatomegaly), nausea (felt to be associated with gastrointestinal wall edema), and leg swelling.

   b. Exam findings suggestive of CHF include jugular venous distension (the vertical distance from the top of the pulsations to the sternal angle), rales or dullness at the lung bases on the pulmonary exam, S3 gallop ($\pm$S4), and dependent lower- extremity edema.

   c. In contrast to acute CHF, the lung exam in chronic CHF may be clear due to lymphatic compensation.

   d. In severe cases of CHF, patients may develop cardiogenic shock, presenting with cool extremities, diaphoresis, tachycardia, and severe dyspnea $\pm$ Cheyne-Stokes respirations. Laboratory values may reflect end-organ damage (elevated creatinine, elevated BUN, decrease in serum sodium, and abnormal liver function tests). Cardiogenic shock requires emergent evaluation by a cardiologist and intensive care unit management.

   e. Diagnostic workup of CHF includes chest X-ray and transthoracic echocardiogram (TTE).

      i. CXR findings include an enlarged heart width (cardiothoracic ratio of >0.5 on posterior–anterior film), upper-zone vascular redistribution (cephalization), pulmonary edema, and pulmonary effusions (right-sided more often than left-sided).

      ii. TTE may show a decreased ejection fraction, an increase in chamber size, and tissue Doppler anomalies.

   f. An elevated brain natriuretic peptide (BNP) may suggest left-sided heart failure. In the clinical setting of CHF, a low to normal BNP may suggest right-sided heart failure, or a noncardiac cause of dyspnea.

   g. Diagnosis and management of CHF in an HSCT patient can be complicated by systemic issues, e.g., concomitant hypoalbuminemia.

h. Management of CHF depends of severity of symptoms and objective findings on TTE; or in severe cases, findings on right-sided cardiac catheterization.

   i. In hemodynamically stable patients with symptoms, management begins with loop diuretics (furosemide) to reduce intravascular volume, angiotensin-converting enzyme (ACE) inhibitors to reverse vasoconstriction, volume retention, ventricular remodeling, and long-acting beta-blockers (carvedilol or metoprolol XL.)

      – Dosing of the loop diuretic may depend on previous exposure to the drug; a "titrate to effect" approach is appropriate. Caution should be used, since over-diuresis may result in acute kidney injury.

   i. Hypoalbuminemia is common in HSCT patients (due to gastrointestinal losses with mucositis, catabolic state, and recognition that albumin is a negative acute-phase reactant) and results in less delivery of loop diuretics to the active site in the kidney. Improvements in diuresis may be effected by titrating an increase in the dose of loop diuretic, initiating a salt-restricted diet or using metolazone (thiazide-like diuretic) to enhance the activity of the loop diuretic. Albumin boluses or infusions have also been used in conjunction with diuretics in this setting to achieve fluid mobilization.

3. Tachyarrhythmias are defined as a heart rate >100 beats per minute for at least 3 beats. Supraventricular tachyarrhythmias (SVT) are typically narrow-complex (narrow QRS) and arise above the ventricles (SVT conducted with aberrancy is an exception), whereas tachyarrhythmias arising within the ventricles typically have wide QRS complexes. Common types of tachyarrhythmias encountered include sinus tachycardia, atrial fibrillation, and atrial flutter. *Sinus tachycardia is extremely common and may not necessarily reflect cardiac dysfunction, but rather other physiologic states, e.g., pain, response to endogenous catecholamines, hypoalbuminemia with third space fluid displacement and intravascular volume depletion.*

   a. Tachyarrhythmias may be perceived as palpitations or light-headedness by the patient. An absence of symptoms is not unusual.

   b. Diagnosis requires capturing a rhythm on ECG or telemetry.

      i. Atrial flutter is characterized by rapid, regular atrial activity at a rate of 150–350 bpm. On EKG, a "saw-toothed" pattern may be seen in lieu of p waves, with breakthrough QRS complexes that appear at a regular or irregular interval.

ii. Atrial fibrillation is a chaotic rhythm without p waves on EKG and erratically occurring QRS complexes, termed "irregularly irregular."

c. Management of tachyarrhythmias includes addressing the underlying cause, which may be circulating cardiac toxins, excess intravascular volume, or intrinsic heart pathology.

  i. In the hemodynamically *unstable* patient, either atrial flutter or atrial fibrillation should be urgently treated with electrical cardioversion.

  ii. The hemodynamically *stable* patient, atrial flutter or atrial fibrillation should be treated by identifying and attempting to reverse the underlying cause.

    – Increases in intravascular volume may stretch the right atrium, triggering a tachyarrhythmia. Diuresis with intravenous loop diuretics is the treatment of choice in this instance.

    – In cases of elevated carbon dioxide levels circulating in the blood, noninvasive positive pressure ventilation may contribute to a reverse of the tachyarrhythmia.

  iii. Stable patients may be treated with electrical cardioversion. The risk of a thrombus in the wall of the heart is lower in the HSCT population compared to the general population, given the concomitant thrombocytopenia.

  iv. Multiple doses of intravenous metoprolol 5 mg IV may be used, typically no more frequent than 3 doses given at 5-min intervals, with close blood pressure monitoring. Long-term rate control may be achieved with oral doses of beta-blockers.

    – Other agents for rate control include digoxin or calcium channel blockers (caution with the latter in cases of impaired ejection fraction.)

20.4 TREATMENT-INDUCED HYPERTENSION

1. Chronic immunosuppression with calcineurin inhibitors (cyclosporine, tacrolimus) following HSCT is a mainstay of therapy for prevention of graft-versus-host disease.

2. Fifteen to fifty percent of patients may develop calcineurin inhibitor-associated hypertension that typically develops within a month of starting treatment; however, may occur later in the treatment course.

3. The treatment of choice is a calcium channel blocker, which reduces peripheral vascular resistance (including the renal arteriolar constriction associated with calcineurin inhibitors) and lowers blood pressure by causing a direct vasodilation in the peripheral arteries of the vascular smooth muscle.

   a. Nifedipine XL 30–60 mg po daily
   b. Amlodipine 2.5–10 mg po daily

4. Posterior reversible encephalopathy syndrome (PRES) is a neurologic complication seen occasionally in patients with calcineurin inhibitor-associated hypertension. The clinical syndrome includes headache, mental status changes, and seizures with specific radiologic features identifiable. Management includes withdrawal of the drug and aggressive control of the hypertension.

20.5 INCIDENCE AND TYPES OF TOXICITIES OCCURRING YEARS FOLLOWING HSCT

1. Long-term survivors of HSCT are more likely to develop diabetes, HTN, dyslipidema, and metabolic syndrome. Cardiovascular outcomes that *do not* occur at an increased incidence include stroke, myocardial infarction, and peripheral vascular disease. Allogeneic HSCT patients have a sevenfold increased risk of a remote cardiovascular event over that of autologous HSCT patients. An increase in remote cardiovascular events may find its origin in vascular dysfunction associated with calcineurin inhibitors, graft-versus-host disease, or direct effects of the transplant procedure. Additionally, chronic GvHD has also been associated with serositis, with clinical presentations of pericardial effusions with tamponade. Finally, iron overload in the post-transplant setting has been associated with chronic cardiac dysfunction. Routine survivorship evaluations screen for systemic iron deposition with recommendations for chelation therapy, when identified (see Chapter 26).

2. In HSCT patients who develop CHF >1 year post-transplant, the average age of onset is 45, suggesting an accelerated course of disease. Risk factors for remote CHF include:

    a. female sex
    b. anthracycline dose >250 mg/m^2 around time of transplant
    c. HTN
    d. acute lung injury
    e. pulmonary HTN
    f. diabetes
3. There are no guidelines to screen for late cardiac complications of HSCT, but adhering to adult screening guidelines for diabetes, hypercholesterolemia, and HTN should be considered a minimum.
4. Currently, there are no available markers to predict the risk of remote CHF.

References

Akahori, M., Nakamae, H., Hino, M., et al. (2003). Electrocardiogram is very useful for predicting acute heart failure following myeloablative chemotherapy with hematopoietic stem cell transplantation rescue. *Bone Marrow Transplant*, 31:585–590.

Armenian, S.H., Sun, C.L., Francisco, L., et al. (2008). Late congestive heart failure after hematopoietic cell transplantation. *J Clin Oncol*, 26:5537–5543.

Baker, K.S., Ness, K.K., Steinberger, J., et al. (2007). Diabetes, hypertension and cardiovascular events in survivors of hematopoietic cell transplantation: A report from the bone marrow transplant survivor study. *Blood*, 109:1765–1772.

Bearman, S.I., Petersen, F.B., Schor, R.A., et al. (1990). Radionuclide ejection fractions in evaluation of patients being considered for bone marrow transplantation. *Bone Marrow Transplant*, 5:173–177.

Cazin, B., Gorin, N.C., Laporte, J.P., et al. (1986). Cardiac complications after bone marrow transplantation. A report on a series of 63 consecutive transplantations. *Cancer*, 57:2061–2069.

Ciresi, D.L., Lloyd, M.A., Sandberg, S.M., et al. (1992). The sodium retaining effects of cyclosporine. *Kidney Int*, 41:1599–1605.

Goldberg, M.A., Antin, J.H., Guinan, E.C., et al. (1986). Cyclophosphamide cardiotoxicity: An analysis of dosing as a risk factor. *Blood*, 68:1114–1118.

Hertenstein, B., Stefanic, M., Scholz, M., et al. (1994). Cardiac toxicity of BMT: Predictive value of cardiologic evaluation before transplant. *J Clin Oncol*, 12:998–1004.

Hildago, J.D., Krone, R., Rich, M.W., et al. (2004). Supraventricular tachyarrhythmias after hematopoietic stem cell transplantation: Incidence, risk factors, and outcomes. *Bone Marrow Transplant*, 34:615–619.

Morandi, P., Ruffini, P.A., Benvenuto, G.M., et al. (2005). Cardiac toxicity of high-dose chemotherapy. *Bone Marrow Transplant*, 35: 323–334.

Murdych, T., Weisdorf, D.J. (2001). Serious cardiac complications during bone marrow transplantation at the University of Minnesota. 1977–1997. *Bone Marrow Transplant*, 28:283–287.

Nakamae, H., Tsumura, K., Hino, M., et al. (2000). QT dispersion as a predictor of acute heart failure after high-dose cyclophosphamide. *Lancet*, 355:805–806.

Rhodes, M., Lautz, T., Kavanaugh-McHugh, A., et al. (2005). Pericardial effusion and cardiac tamponade in pediatric stem cell transplant recipients. *Bone Marrow Transplant*, 36:139–144.

Sakata-Yanagimoto, M., Kanda, Y., Nakagawa, M., et al. (2004). Predictors for severe cardiac complications after hematopoietic stem cell transplantation. *Bone Marrow Transplant*, 33:1043–1047.

Santos, G.W., Senbrenner, L.L., Bruke, P.J. et al. (1972). The use of cyclophosphamide for clinical marrow transplantation. *Transplant Proc*, 4:559–564.

Tichelli, A., Bucher, C, Rovo, A., et al. (2007). Premature cardiovascular disease after allogeneic hematopoietic stem cell transplant. *Blood*, 110:3463–3471.

Tang, W.H.W., Thomas, S., Kalaycio, M., et al. (2004). Clinical outcomes of patients with impaired left ventricular ejection fraction undergoing autologous bone marrow transplantation: Can we safely transplant patients with impaired ejection fraction? *Bone Marrow Transplant*, 34:603–607.

CHAPTER 21
Acute Kidney Injury

Anuja Mittalhenkle

Renal complications including acute kidney injury (AKI) and chronic kidney disease (CKD) are important complications following hematopoietic stem cell transplantation (HSCT). AKI requiring renal replacement therapy (RRT) in critically ill HSCT patients is associated with a poor prognosis. Mortality for patients receiving myeloablative allogeneic HSCTs who require dialysis exceeds 80%.

21.1 DEFINITIONS OF AKI AND CKD

1. AKI (previously acute renal failure or ARF): There is still no consensus definition for AKI, but most staging systems use increase in serum creatinine or decrease in urine output. AKI criteria include more than 1.5-fold increase in creatinine from baseline or oliguria (urine output <0.5 mL/kg/h for more than 6 h). Diagnosis of AKI may be missed in HSCT patients. In HSCT patients who have cachexia and low muscle mass, the baseline creatinine may be abnormally low. Also, patients who are on diuretics may maintain urine output due to medications, but have already reduced glomerular filtration rate (GFR).

2. CKD: CKD is defined as evidence of kidney abnormalities (structural or functional) that persist for at least 3 months. Reduced GFR and persistent albuminuria are the most common manifestations of chronic kidney injury. Five stages of CKD are defined based on GFR (see Table 21.1).

R.T. Maziarz, S. Slater (eds.), *Blood and Marrow Transplant Handbook*, DOI 10.1007/978-1-4419-7506-5_21, © Springer Science+Business Media, LLC 2011

TABLE 21.1. Stages of CKD

Stage	GFR (mL/min/1.73 m^2)
1	>90
2	60–89
3	30–59
4	15–29
5	<15

21.2 INCIDENCE OF AKI

The incidence of renal injury is influenced by the type of HSCT performed.

1. Myeloablative allogeneic HSCT: Incidence of AKI is highest after myeloablative allogeneic transplant. Incidence of moderate to severe renal failure, defined as doubling of serum creatinine, has ranged from 36 to 78% with 20–33% requiring renal replacement therapy (RRT).
2. Nonmyeloablative allogeneic HSCT: About 30–40% of patients develop moderate to severe renal failure, with ~4% requiring RRT. Many of these patients also have baseline chronic kidney disease, as they tend to be older than other HSCT patients.
3. Autologous HSCT: Incidence of renal failure is lowest in this patient population with ~20% incidence, with reports as high as 7% for patients in need of RRT.

21.3 GENERAL CLASSIFICATION OF CAUSES AND BASIC WORKUP OF AKI

It is useful to consider causes as prerenal, intrinsic renal, and postrenal in order to have a systematic approach to evaluating a patient with acute kidney injury.

1. Prerenal causes include volume depletion (vomiting, diarrhea, poor fluid intake), sinusoidal obstruction syndrome (veno-occlusive disease), drugs (CSA, tacrolimus)
2. Intrinsic renal causes include acute tubular necrosis (ATN) due to ischemia or sepsis, IV contrast induced, thrombotic microangiopathy
3. Postrenal causes include intrarenal obstruction from uric acid , extrarenal obstruction from bladder outlet obstruction (e.g., narcotics, clot from hemorrhagic cystitis)

4. Basic renal tests that may be useful
   a. urinalysis
   b. spot urine for sodium
   c. protein and creatinine
   d. bladder scan (to check post-void residual)
   e. renal ultrasound to look at kidney and bladder

21.4 TIMING AND CAUSE OF RENAL INJURY

1. Induction therapy
   a. tumor lysis syndrome
   b. marrow infusion toxicity
2. Weeks post-HSCT
   a. volume depletion
   b. sinusoidal obstruction syndrome (SOS)
   c. medications (e.g., calcineurin inhibitors, antibiotics, antivirals, amphotericin products)
   d. acute tubular necrosis (ATN)
   e. hemorrhagic cystitis
   f. thrombotic microangiopathy
3. Months post-HSCT
   a. calcineurin inhibitor
   b. thrombotic microangiopathy

21.5 EVALUATION AND MANAGEMENT OF COMMON CAUSES OF RENAL INJURY

It is important to prevent renal injury if possible, given the high rate of mortality associated with renal failure requiring dialysis. This can be achieved by closely monitoring renal function, avoiding nephrotoxic agents when feasible, and appropriately dosing medications for level of renal function. Adequate hydration, as is standard with chemotherapy protocols, is important. Consulting a nephrology specialist early in the course of AKI, rather than waiting until renal replacement therapy is imminent, is recommended.

1. Tumor lysis syndrome (TLS) is caused by tumor cell lysis and results in hyperuricemia, hyperphosphatemia, hyperkalemia, and hypocalcemia with subsequent acute kidney injury.
   a. Mechanism of renal injury: Hyperuricemia leads to increased excretion of uric acid, precipitation of uric

acid in the renal tubules and toxicity to renal epithelial and endothelial cells. Hyperphosphatemia can lead to intrarenal deposition of calcium phosphate crystals and direct toxicity to tubules.

b. Prophylaxis

i. Intravenous fluids: Aggressive intravenous hydration is important to establish high urine output to prevent precipitation of uric acid in the renal tubules in intermediate- and high-risk patients. Guidelines recommend solution of 5% dextrose one quarter normal saline as IVF for both pediatric and adult patients and normal (isotonic) saline if patients are volume depleted or hyponatremic.

ii. Allopurinol: Decreases formation of new uric acid by blocking the metabolism of xanthine to uric acid. The usual dose in adults is 100 mg/m^2 every 8 h. The maximum dose is 800 mg per day and dose must be reduced in renal failure. It is started 1–2 days prior to induction chemotherapy and continued for up to 7 days after the tumor lysis labs have become normal.

iii. Recombinant urate oxidase (Rasburicase®): Lowers uric acid (including preformed uric acid) by increasing the conversion of uric acid to water soluble allantoin. It can be used for both preventing and treating hyperuricemia. Recommended dose is 0.15–0.2 mg/kg in 50 mL of isotonic saline over 30 min daily for 5 days, but lower doses may be effective in some patients. Specific institutional guidelines are often established for administration of rasburicase.

c. Management

i. Hyperuricemia: Give Rasburicase if not already given.

ii. Hyperkalemia: Check EKG and give calcium gluconate for reducing cardiac toxicity. Potassium can be shifted into the intracellular compartment by using insulin and glucose. It is important to make sure that the patient is on a low-potassium diet and no exogenous potassium is being given in IV fluids or oral supplementation. In order to remove potassium, loop diuretics, kayexalate, or dialysis is needed. Potassium level >6.0 can become life-threatening, and appropriate treatment must be instituted promptly.

iii. Hyperphosphatemia: Patients should be put on a low-phosphate diet and an oral phosphate binder started with meals. Unless the patient is symptomatic from hypocalcemia, avoid giving calcium supplementation in order to avoid precipitation of calcium phosphate crystals in the kidney. Dialysis may be required. Examples of phosphate binders include:

- Aluminum hydroxide can be given orally at 50–150 mg/kg/day divided into three or four doses/day with meals to bind dietary phosphorus in the GI tract. Due to concern for aluminum toxicity, this binder should be used for a short duration only (1–2 days).
- Calcium containing formulations (calcium carbonate and acetate)
- Sevelamer hydroxide 800–1,600 mg with each meal depending on serum phosphorus level
- Lanthanum carbonate 1,500–3,000 mg po daily in divided doses.

iv. Hypocalcemia: Give IV calcium only if patient has symptoms. In patients with severe symptoms such as cardiac arrhythmias and tetany, IV calcium gluconate should be given even if patient has hyperphosphatemia.

v. AKI: Supportive care is needed, which includes avoiding nephrotoxic drugs and IV contrast, dosing medications for renal function, and managing volume status. Nephrology specialist should be consulted if electrolyte abnormalities persist, hyperuricemia is not responsive to interventions, or patient is oliguric. Hemodialysis or continuous renal replacement therapy may be needed for uric acid and phosphate clearance.

2. Marrow infusion toxicity can occur in patients undergoing autologous HSCT. DMSO, a cryopreservative, can cause in vivo hemolysis, which can lead to pigment nephropathy and AKI. This is a rare complication now with changes in preservation techniques for stem cells.

3. Sepsis: Neutropenia is the predisposing factor in HSCT patients. Renal injury occurs due to renal hypoperfusion, which is a result of vasodilation and capillary leak. Cytokines induce inflammation and vasoconstriction in the kidney. Antibiotics used for prevention or treatment of infections can further exacerbate the AKI. Supportive care is needed if AKI develops along with treatment of the underlying infection. A Transplant Infectious Disease consult can be

helpful in choosing appropriate drugs that may be less nephrotoxic.

4. Sinusoidal obstruction syndrome (SOS): This syndrome is a result of conditioning therapy injuring endothelial cells of hepatic venules. This leads to thrombosis of small vessels, resulting in sinusoidal and portal hypertension. Patients develop a sodium avid state, which leads to weight gain and peripheral edema. Patients also manifest painful hepatomegaly and jaundice. Subsequently, urea and creatinine start rising and urinary sodium is low, despite use of diuretics. Patients can become volume overloaded as they have high fluid intake (medications, nutrition, etc.) and poor response to diuretics. Dialysis may be required to manage volume overload and worsening azotemia.

5. Drug toxicity: Many drugs used in HSCT are nephrotoxic. These include chemotherapy agents (methotrexate), antimicrobial agents (Amphotericin B, aminoglycosides), and immunosuppressants (cyclosporine, tacrolimus). Liposomal formulations of Amphotericin are considered to have lower nephrotoxicity. Appropriately timed drug levels should be checked if an aminoglycoside or vancomycin is used to avoid or reduce renal injury.

6. Calcineurin inhibitors (CNI): Cyclosporine and tacrolimus are used for prophylaxis for graft-versus-host disease (GvHD). Both drugs are vasoconstricting and nephrotoxic. Trough drug levels should be monitored and dose should be reduced or drug temporarily held if a patient develops AKI. CNI can lead to chronic kidney disease, and have been implicated in cases of thrombotic microangiopathy (see Chapter 22).

7. Thrombotic microangiopathy (TMA): Seen late in HSCT and can lead to chronic kidney disease. This has been reported in 15–20% of survivors of allogeneic HSCT. TMA may be the result of the conditioning regimen, GvHD, or infection. Presentation includes hematuria, proteinuria, hypertension, and renal failure. Patients have microangiopathic anemia, with elevated LDH, decreased haptoglobin, and thrombocytopenia. Both the thrombotic microangiopathy and resultant hemoglobinuria cause acute tubular necrosis (ATN). TMA-related renal failure requires supportive therapy. Plasma exchange in HSCT-related TMA may not have the same success rates as in renal failure due to TMA from other causes. Some patients have renal recovery but many develop CKD.

8. Nephrotic Syndrome: Patients present with proteinuria (usually >3.5 g/24 h), hypoalbuminemia, and edema. Many patients have membranous nephropathy on renal biopsy, which may be a manifestation of chronic graft-versus-host disease (GVHD) in the kidney. Minimal change disease, IgA nephropathy, focal segmental glomerulosclerosis (FSGS), and ANCA-associated glomerulonephritis have also been reported. Patients have been treated with high-dose steroids, cyclosporine, and other immunosuppressive agents to achieve resolution of the nephrotic syndrome.

References

Ando, M., Ohashi, K., Akiyama, H., Sakamaki, H., Morito, T., Tsuchiya, K., et al. (2010). Chronic kidney disease in long-term survivors of myeloablative allogeneic hematopoietic cell transplantation: Prevalence and risk factors. *Nephrol Dial Transplant, 25*: 278–282.

Coiffier, B., Altman, A., Pui, C.H., Younes, A., Cairo, M.S. (2008). Guidelines for the management of pediatric and adult tumor lysis syndrome: An evidence-based review. *J Clin Oncol, 26*:2767–2778.

Colombo, A.A., Rusconi, C., Esposito, C., Bernasconi, P., Caldera, D., Lazzarino, M., et al. (2006). Nephrotic syndrome after allogeneic hematopoietic stem cell transplantation as a late complication of chronic graft-versus-host disease. *Transplantation, 81*:1087–1092.

Ellis, M.J., Parikh, C.R., Inrig, J.K., Kanbay, M., Patel, U.D. (2008). Chronic kidney disease after hematopoietic cell transplantation: A systematic review. *Am J Transplant, 8*:2378–2390.

Herget-Rosenthal, S., Uppenkamp, M., Beelen, D., Kohl, D., Kribben, A. (2000). Renal complications of high-dose chemotherapy and peripheral blood stem cell transplantation. *Nephron, 84*:136–141.

Hingorani, S. (2006). Chronic kidney disease in long-term survivors of hematopoietic cell transplantation: Epidemiology, pathogenesis, and treatment. *J Am Soc Nephrol, 17*:1995–2005.

Hingorani, S.R., Guthrie, K., Batchelder, A., Schoch, G., Aboulhosn, N., Manchion, J., et al. (2005). Acute renal failure after myeloablative hematopoietic cell transplant: Incidence and risk factors. *Kidney Int, 67*:272–277.

Humphreys, B.D., Soiffer, R.J., Magee, C.C. (2005). Renal failure associated with cancer and its treatment: An update. *J Am Soc Nephrol, 16*:151–161.

Kersting, S., Dorp, S.V., Theobald, M., Verdonck, L.F. (2008). Acute renal failure after nonmyeloablative stem cell transplantation in adults. *Bio Blood Marrow Transplant, 14*:125–131.

Lameire, N., van Biesen, W., Vanholder, R. (2008). Acute renal problems in the critically ill cancer patient. *Curr Opin Crit Care, 14*:635–646.

Parikh, C.R., Schrier, R.W., Storer, B., Diaconescu, R., Sorror, M.L., Maris, M.B., et al. (2005). Comparison of ARF after myeloablative and nonmyeloablative hematopoietic cell transplantation. *Am J Kidney Dis, 45*:502–509.

Parikh, C.R., McSweeney, P., Schrier, R.W. (2005). Acute renal failure independently predicts mortality after myeloablative allogeneic hematopoietic cell transplant. *Kidney Int, 67*:1999–2005.

Parikh, C.R., Coca, S.G. (2006). Acute renal failure in hematopoietic cell transplantation. *Kidney Int, 69*:430–435.

Touzot, M., Elie, C., van Massenhove, J., Maillard, N., Buzyn, A., Fakhourt, F. (2010). Long-term renal function after allogeneic haematopoietic stem cell transplantation in adult patients: A single-centre study. *Nephrol Dial Transplant, 25*:624–627.

Troxell, M.L., Pilapil, M., Miklos, D.B., Higgins, J.P., Kambham, N. (2008). Renal pathology in hematopoietic cell transplantation recipients. *Mod Pathol. 21*:396–406.

Zager, R.A. (1994). Acute renal failure in the setting of bone marrow transplantation. *Kidney Int, 46*:1443–1458.

Zager, R.A., O'Quigley, J., Zager, B.K., Alpers, C.E., Shulman, H.M., Gamelin, L.M., et al. (1989). Acute renal failure following bone marrow transplantation: a retrospective study of 272 patients. *Am J Kidney Dis, 13*:210–216.

CHAPTER 22
Thrombotic Microangiopathies

Thomas DeLoughery

The thrombotic microangiopathies (TMs) are a group of diseases that share the qualities of thrombocytopenia and microangiopathic hemolytic anemia resulting in microvascular occlusion and end-organ damage. The "classic" TMs are thrombotic thrombocytopenic purpura (TTP) and hemolytic uremic syndrome (HUS). Since the early days of transplantation, it has been noted many patients developed a TM-type disease that was often fulminant and fatal. Research has been difficult due to lack of standardization of diagnostic criteria, and much controversy remains about the best therapy.

22.1 CLINICAL PRESENTATION

The basic problem in all TMs is occlusion of the vasculature by platelet aggregates. This event restricts blood flow, which leads to areas of high shear that damage red cells leading to fragmentation. This is the origin of the "helmet cells" or "schistocytes" part of the diagnostic criteria ("microangiopathic hemolytic anemia"). The vascular occlusion leads to tissue ischemia and end-organ damage. In classic HUS, this pathophysiology is restricted to the kidney leading to renal failure, while in TTP it can occur in any organ. The high LDH that is seen in TM is due both to red cell destruction and to tissue ischemia. In transplant patients, the onset of the TM is often gradual, with slowly rising LDH and deteriorating renal function. In TM associated with agents such as calcineurin inhibitors, the onset can be more rapid. As the TM progresses, renal insufficiency and neurological symptoms are the most common findings, in many patients running a relentless course until the patient expires.

R.T. Maziarz, S. Slater (eds.), *Blood and Marrow Transplant Handbook*, DOI 10.1007/978-1-4419-7506-5_22, © Springer Science+Business Media, LLC 2011

22.2 RISK FACTORS

Many risk factors for TM have been proposed. One difficulty with these risk factors is that any widespread disease process such as severe infections or GvHD can lead to a clinical syndrome similar to TM. This lack of clarity in identification of etiologic events results in the extreme variations in reported incidence rates ranging from 0 to 93% of patients.

Risk factors include:

1. Older age
2. Female gender
3. Advanced disease
4. Unrelated donor transplant
5. Irradiation-containing preparative regimens
6. Use of calcineurin inhibitors
7. Infections
8. GvHD

22.3 CLASSIFICATION

Pettit and Clark in 1994 proposed a classification that still provides a useful schema for thinking about transplant-related TM.

1. One group is the "multi-organ fulminant," which occurs early (20–60 days), has multi-organ system involvement, and is often fatal.
2. A second type of TTP/HUS is similar to cyclosporine/tacrolimus HUS.
3. A third type described as "conditioning" TTP/HUS occurs 6 months or more after total body irradiation and is associated with primary renal involvement.
4. Finally, patients with systemic CMV infections may present with a TTP/HUS syndrome related to vascular infection with CMV.

22.4 ETIOLOGY

In classic TTP, most patients have very low levels of ADAMTS-13 (<5%), which is thought to lead to spontaneous platelet aggregation via the failure to cleave the ultra-high molecular weight multimers of von Willebrand protein. In patients with transplant-related TM, most reports show reduced but not extremely low levels of ADAMTS-13. The underlying factor in most transplant-associated TMs is endothelial damage, either by GvHD, medications, irradiation, or infection. This endothelial damage leads to platelet aggregation, microangiopathic hemolytic anemia, and end-organ damage. This premise that endothelial damage is the main trigger for transplant TM would explain why many of the risk factors for TM share the fact they involve vascular damage.

22.5 DIAGNOSIS

Given that the diagnosis of any TM is a clinical one and that transplant patients are prone to have many complications that can mimic a TM, it is easy to appreciate and understand the great center-to-center variation in describing the incidence. Recently, two groups have proposed diagnostic consensus criteria that share the common features of evidence of a microangiopathic hemolytic anemia and elevated LDH. However, applying these criteria to an individual patient still requires clinical judgment.

1. Blood and Marrow Transplant Clinical Trial Network (BMTCTN) Criteria
   a. RBC fragmentation and ≥ 2 schistocytes per high-powered field
   b. Concurrent increase in LDH from institutional baseline
   c. Concurrent renal and/or neurological dysfunction with no other explanation
   d. Negative Coombs test
2. International Working Group Criteria
   a. Increased percentage (>4%) of schistocytes in the blood
   b. New, prolonged, or progressive thrombocytopenia (<50,000/μL or >50% decrease from previous counts)
   c. Sudden and persistent increase in LDH
   d. Decreased hemoglobin or increased transfusion requirements
   e. Decrease in serum haptoglobin

22.6 TREATMENT

1. Cyclosporine/tacrolimus TM: This often occurs either days after the introduction of these medications or with an increase in blood levels of these agents. The renal and neurological manifestation can be rapid and severe, including malignant hypertension, seizures, and cortical blindness. Therapy is discontinuation of the medications and to

manage the closely associated hypertension. In patients with mild TM and high serum levels, one can lower the dose to see if the symptoms abate.

2. Conditioning TM: This is rare and may be a manifestation of radiation damage to the vasculature. Usually, the course is progressive with no specific therapy available.

3. Systemic CMV TM: CMV is trophic to the endothelium, and aggressive therapy of CMV is the cornerstone of therapy.

4. Multi-organ fulminant: Therapy remains unsatisfactory. The first step is to maximize treatment of any process that may be aggravating the TM (GvHD, infections, etc.). Unlike classic TTP, the role of plasma exchange remains controversial. Most series report very poor response rates and outcomes with high rates of complications. Commonly, the patient may respond for a few days but then relapse. A practical approach would be to use one plasma volume/day exchange in patients with TM until it is clear they are not responding to therapy.

References

Batts, E.D., Lazarus, H.M. (2007). Diagnosis and treatment of transplantation-associated thrombotic microangiopathy: Real progress or are we still waiting? *Bone Marrow Transplant*, 40:709–719.

Ho, V.T., Cutler, C., Carter, S., Martin, P., Adams, R., Horowitz, M., et al. (2005). Blood and marrow transplant clinical trials network toxicity committee consensus summary: Thrombotic microangiopathy after hematopoietic stem cell transplantation. *Biol Blood Marrow Transplant*, 11:571–575.

Pettitt, A.R., Clark, R.E. (1994) Thrombotic microangiopathy following bone marrow transplantation. *Bone Marrow Transplant*, 14: 495–504.

Ruutu, T., Barosi, G., Benjamin, R.J., Clark, R.E., George, J.N., Gratwohl, A. et al. (2007). European Group for blood and marrow transplantation; European LeukemiaNet. Diagnostic criteria for hematopoietic stem cell transplant-associated microangiopathy: Results of a consensus process by an International Working Group. *Haematologica*, 92:95–100.

CHAPTER 23
Graft Failure

Gabrielle Meyers

The failure to establish hematopoiesis after hematopoietic stem cell transplantation (HSCT) is a devastating complication that can occur during both autologous and allogeneic stem cell transplant. Early graft failure carries a poor prognosis; patients who develop late graft failure generally do slightly better. Numerous factors are known to increase the risk of engraftment failure; and working to reduce the risk upfront to minimize this tragic complication is vital, as despite improvements in supportive care the mortality associated with primary engraftment failure remains very high. In the setting of autologous stem cell transplant, newer agents to enhance mobilization of stem cells and recognition of clear minimum stem cell doses required to proceed with the procedure have minimized the risks of graft failure as best as possible. However, in the allogeneic transplant setting, a combination of factors has made graft failure a continued concern. Integration of high-resolution HLA typing has reduced the risk of graft failure over the past decades; yet with the ever increasing use of nonmyeloablative conditioning regimens and alternative graft options, this complication remains an issue. Optimal antibody testing of donors and recipients prior to transplant, choice of product and dose, and enhanced use of immunosuppressive agents as part of the conditioning regimen may minimize the risk of engraftment failure. In addition, prompt recognition of those at highest risk of engraftment failure and rapid steps to collect additional product provide the best chance of salvaging patients from complications of prolonged and profound pancytopenia.

R.T. Maziarz, S. Slater (eds.), *Blood and Marrow Transplant Handbook*, DOI 10.1007/978-1-4419-7506-5_23, © Springer Science+Business Media, LLC 2011

23.1 AUTOLOGOUS TRANSPLANT

1. Engraftment failure is defined as a failure to achieve an absolute neutrophil count of 200/mm^3 by day +21. Hematopoietic recovery may be transient, partial, or absent
2. From an immunological standpoint, graft rejection is not considered possible, but graft failure (non-engraftment) may still be seen.
3. Graft failure may be the consequence of
   a. infusion of an inadequate number of stem cells
   b. a damaged marrow microenvironment
   c. concomitant infections, e.g., CMV
   d. cryopreservation techniques that may damage stem cells
   e. post-transplant medications, e.g., trimethoprim/sulfamethoxazole or ganciclovir

23.2 ALLOGENEIC TRANSPLANT

1. It is critical to differentiate between graft failure and graft rejection.
   a. Primary engraftment failure is defined as a complete lack of engraftment (absolute neutrophil count <500/mm^3 without evidence of relapse) by day +28 post-transplant, irrespective of source of stem cells.
   b. Late graft failure is defined as development of pancytopenia and marrow aplasia later after transplant in the setting of previous establishment of donor-derived hematopoiesis.
   c. Graft rejection is best defined by the demonstration of donor chimerism that diminishes over time, in parallel with the development of peripheral cytopenias. This can best be monitored by following donor lymphocyte pools. Persistence of host-derived cytotoxic T cells or NK cells or initiation of a GVH reaction from donor cells may also lead to failure to maintain the stem cell graft.
2. HLA antibody screening pre-transplant is a highly useful tool to assess for donor-directed HLA-specific allo-antibodies, which are known to markedly increase the risk of graft failure, particularly in the setting of partially matched or mismatched transplants.
   a. Determination of a positive panel reactive antibody (PRA) necessitates further investigation to determine HLA specificities.
   b. The finding of donor-directed HLA-specific alloantibodies markedly increases the risk of graft failure and must be strongly considered in donor selection.

23.3 DONOR LEUKOCYTE INFUSION

Donor leukocyte infusions (DLI) are a frequently utilized strategy for patients who relapse after allogeneic transplantation.

1. DLI infusion(s) may result in a significant degree of myelosuppression and even aplasia. It is hypothesized that aplasia is due to T-cells that are transfused in the donor leukocyte product recognizing residual host marrow cells and destroying them.
2. If the patient has severe chronic GvHD or minimal residual donor cells are detected in the pre-DLI chimerism studies, hematopoiesis may not recover without the infusion of donor hematopoietic stem cells in the donor leukocyte product.

23.4 RISK FACTORS FOR GRAFT FAILURE

1. HLA-incompatible graft
2. Matched unrelated donor graft
3. Cord blood donor graft
4. Aplastic anemia (in particular, heavily transfused pre-transplant)
5. Fanconi anemia, thalassemia, or immunodeficiency diagnoses
6. Inadequate or limited pre-transplant conditioning regimen
7. T-cell depletion or ex vivo purging
8. Infections (CMV-positive recipient in particular)
9. Cell dose <2.0 × 10^9/kg
10. Myelotoxins
11. Damaged marrow microenvironment
12. Allosensitization

23.5 DIAGNOSIS

1. Peripheral blood cell counts. Of note, previous studies have shown that a leukocyte count of <200/microliter on day +16 post-transplant is a strong predictor of subsequent primary graft failure.
2. Bone marrow aspirate and biopsy
   a. In both autologous and allogeneic patients, bone marrow studies show a hypocellular marrow with no identifiable myeloid, erythroid, or megakaryocytic precursor cells.
3. FISH/cytogenetics for sex chromosomes or disease-specific double fusion products (i.e., BCR/abl)

4. Variable number of tandem repeats (**VNTR**) is a molecular diagnostic test used to determine post-transplant engraftment/chimerism. These studies require pre-transplant storage of blood (DNA material) from both donor and recipient. It is most useful in same sex transplants where FISH for XX and XY is not applicable.
5. Infectious disease testing, specifically CMV PCR, HHV6 PCR

23.6 TREATMENT

1. Hematopoietic growth factors (e.g., GM-CSF) are more successful in the setting of hematopoietic failure.
2. Stem cell boost (±additional conditioning agents), i.e., backup stem cell/marrow infusion, second transplant, etc. There are multiple case reports and studies showing successful engraftment after the use of fludarabine ± low-dose TBI-containing regimens prior to infusion of more product.
3. Immunosuppression particularly in this setting of failing donor chimerism.
4. Pharmocologic review to remove myelotoxins (ganciclovir, ACE inhibitors, bactrim, vancomycin, linezolid, H_2 blockers, etc.).
5. Eliminate infections.
6. Consider dose escalated G-CSF 10 mcg/kg/day vs. 5 mcg/kg BID.

References

Ahmed, N., Leung, K.S., Rosenblatt, H., Bollard, C.M., Gottschalk, S., Myers, G.D., et al. (2008). Successful treatment of stem cell graft failure in pediatric patients using a submyeloablative regimen of campath-1H and fludarabine. *Biol Blood Marrow Transplant*, 14: 1298–1304.

Byrne, B.J., Horwitz, M., Long, G.D., Gasparetto, C., Sullivan, K.M., Chute, J., et al. (2008). Outcomes of a second non-myeloablative allogeneic stem cell transplantation following graft rejection. *Bone Marrow Transplant*, 41:39–43.

Champlin, R.E., Horowitz, M.M., van Bekkum, D.W., Camitta, B.M., Elfenbein, G.E., Gale, R.P., et al. (1989). Graft failure following bone marrow transplantation for severe aplastic anemia: Risk factors and treatment results. *Blood*, 73:606–613.

Chan, K.W., Grimley, M.S., Taylor, C., Wall, D.A. (2008). Early identification and management of graft failure after unrelated cord blood transplantation. *Bone Marrow Transplant*, 42:35–41.

Chewning, J.H., Castro-Malaspina, H., Jakubowski, A., Kernan, N.A., Papadopoulos, E.B., Small, T.N., et al. (2007). Fludarabine-based conditioning secures engraftment of second hematopoietic stem cell allografts (HSCT) in the treatment of initial graft failure. *Biol Blood Marrow Transplant*, 13:1313–1323.

Ciurea, S.O., de Lima, M., Cano, P., Korbling, M., Giralt, S., Shpall, E.J., et al. (2009). High risk of graft failure in patients with anti-HLA antibodies undergoing haploidentical stem-cell transplantation. *Transplantation*, 88:1019–1024.

Dvorak, C.C., Gilman, A.L., Horn, B., Cowan, M.J. (2009) Primary graft failure after umbilical cord blood transplant rescued by parental haplocompatible stem cell transplantation. *J Pediatr Hematol Oncol*, 31:300–303.

Grandage, V.L., Cornish, J.M., Pamphilon, D.H., Potter, M.N., Steward, C.G., Oakhill, A., et al. (1998). Second allogeneic bone marrow transplants from unrelated donors for graft failure following initial unrelated donor bone marrow transplantation. *Bone Marrow Transplant*, 21:687–690.

Guardiola, P., Kuentz, M., Garban, F., Blaise, D., Reiffers, J., Attal, M., et al. (2000). Second early allogeneic stem cell transplantations for graft failure in acute leukaemia, chronic myeloid leukaemia and aplastic anaemia. French Society of Bone Marrow Transplantation. *Br J Haematol*, 111:292–302.

Gutman, J.A., McKinney, S.K., Pereira, S., Warnock, S.L., Smith, A.G., Woolfrey, A.E., et al. (2009). Prospective monitoring for alloimmunization in cord blood transplantation: "virtual crossmatch" can be used to demonstrate donor-directed antibodies. *Transplantation*, 87:415–418.

Jabbour, E., Rondon, G., Anderlini, P., Giralt, S.A., Couriel, D.R., Champlin, R.E., et al. (2007). Treatment of donor graft failure with nonmyeloablative conditioning of fludarabine, antithymocyte globulin and a second allogeneic hematopoietic transplantation. *Bone Marrow Transplant*, 40:431–435.

Mattsson, J., Ringdén, O., Storb, R. (2008). Graft failure after allogeneic hematopoietic cell transplantation. *Biol Blood Marrow Transplant*, 14(Suppl 1), 165–170.

McCann, S.R., Bacigalupo, A., Gluckman, E., Hinterberger, W., Hows, J., Ljungman, P., et al. (1994). Graft rejection and second bone marrow transplants for acquired aplastic anaemia: A report from the Aplastic Anaemia Working Party of the European Bone Marrow Transplant Group. *Bone Marrow Transplant*, 13:233–237.

Mehta, J., Powles, R., Singhal, S., Horton, C., Middleton, G., Eisen, T., et al. (1997). Early identification of patients at risk of death due to infections, hemorrhage, or graft failure after allogeneic bone marrow transplantation on the basis of the leukocyte counts. *Bone Marrow Transplant*, 19:349–355.

Nemunaitis, J., Singer, J.W., Buckner, C.D., Durnam, D., Epstein, C., Hill, R., et al. (1990). Use of recombinant human granulocyte-macrophage colony-stimulating factor in graft failure after bone marrow transplantation. *Blood*, 76:245–253.

Platzbecker, U., Binder, M., Schmid, C., Rutt, C., Ehninger, G., Bornhäuser, M. (2008). Second donation of hematopoietic stem cells from unrelated donors for patients with relapse or graft failure after allogeneic transplantation. *Haematologica*, 93:1276–1278.

Pottinger, B., Walker, M., Campbell, M., Holyoake, T.L., Franklin, I.M., Cook, G. (2002). The storage and re-infusion of autologous blood and BM as back-up following failed primary hematopoietic stem-cell transplantation: A survey of European practice. *Cytotherapy*, 4:127–135.

Remberger, M., Ringdén, O., Ljungman, P., Hägglund, H., Winiarski, J., Lönnqvist, B., et al. (1998). Booster marrow or blood cells for graft failure after allogeneic bone marrow transplantation. *Bone Marrow Transplant*, 22:73–78.

Rondón, G., Saliba, R.M., Khouri, I., Giralt, S., Chan, K., Jabbour, E., et al. (2008). Long-term follow-up of patients who experienced graft failure postallogeneic progenitor cell transplantation. Results of a single institution analysis. *Biol Blood Marrow Transplant*, 14: 859–866.

Schriber, J., Agovi, M.A., Ho, V., Ballen, K.K., Bacigalupo, A., Lazarus, H.M., et al. (2010). Second unrelated donor hematopoietic cell transplantation for primary graft failure. *Biol Blood Marrow Transplant*, 16:1099–1106.

Spellman, S., Bray, R., Rosen-Bronson, S., Haagenson, M., Klein, J., Flesch, S., et al. (2010). The detection of donor-directed, HLA-specific alloantibodies in recipients of unrelated hematopoietic cell transplantation is predictive of graft failure. *Blood*, 115:2704–2708.

Stellje, M., van Biezen, A., Slavin, S., Olavarria, E., Clark, R.E., Nagler, A., et al. (2008). The harvest and use of autologous back-up grafts for graft failure or severe GVHD after allogeneic hematopoietic stem cell transplantation: A survey of the European Group for Blood and Marrow Transplantation. *Bone Marrow Transplant*, 42:739–742.

Weisdorf, D.J., Verfaillie, C.M., Davies, S.M., Filipovich, A.H., Wagner, J.E. Jr, Miller, J.S., et al. (1995). Hematopoietic growth factors for graft failure after bone marrow transplantation: A randomized trial of granulocyte-macrophage colony-stimulating factor (GM-CSF) versus sequential GM-CSF plus granulocyte-CSF. *Blood*, 85:3452–3456.

CHAPTER 24
Post-transplant Relapse

Richard T. Maziarz and Susan Slater

Despite the advances in the field of stem cell transplantation, relapse remains a major source of mortality. CIBMTR data identify relapse as the cause of death in 78% of autologous transplant patients, 34% of related allogeneic transplant patients, and 23% of unrelated transplant patients. With the advent of reduced intensity transplants allowing more patients to proceed with transplant, there have been reports of higher than anticipated relapses. Management of relapse post-transplant requires assessment of multiple host/recipient factors and often is limited by the compromised status of the recipient.

In 2008, the National Cancer Institute hosted a meeting at the annual conference of the American Society of Hematology, which led to the creation of subcommittees tasked with addressing the biology, epidemiology, prevention, monitoring, and treatment of relapsed disease. Each committee reviewed the available scientific data and identified areas of research to be pursued. Publication of these results and recommendations in the *Biology of Blood and Marrow Transplantation* began in May, 2010, and will continue over the course of the following months.

24.1 CONSIDERATIONS FOR AUTOLOGOUS TRANSPLANT RECIPIENTS

1. Autologous transplantation is offered to patients with either curative intent or with the goal of improved progression-free survival.

R.T. Maziarz, S. Slater (eds.), *Blood and Marrow Transplant Handbook*, DOI 10.1007/978-1-4419-7506-5_24, © Springer Science+Business Media, LLC 2011

2. The interval between transplant and relapse/progression can be predictive of likelihood of success of retreatment.
3. Options for administration of chemotherapy with therapeutic intent post-autologous transplantation can be limited due to poor marrow reserve.
4. Allogeneic transplantation is often considered as a treatment option for patients who relapse after autologous transplantation.
5. Lenalidomide maintenance therapy has been shown to increase progression-free survival in patients with multiple myeloma status post autologous transplantation; randomized trials assessing maintenance therapy after autologous transplantation for non-Hodgkin lymphoma have been performed and results of data analysis are pending.

24.2 CONSIDERATIONS FOR ALLOGENEIC TRANSPLANT RECIPIENTS

1. The decision to pursue post-relapse therapy is influenced by the interval from transplant to relapse, the clinical condition of the patient, the presence or absence of active GvHD, and the kinetics of the disease recurrence
2. Indolent relapse is more likely to be successfully treated with manipulations of the donor immune system
3. Aggressive relapse often requires chemotherapy administration resulting in a CR or near CR of the hematologic malignancy prior to immunologic manipulation
4. Withdrawal of immune suppression to stimulate a graft-vs-leukemia effect requires confirmation of absence of active GvHD
5. Chemotherapy and/or donor leukocyte infusions (DLI)
   a. DLI has been proven to be most successful in patients with CML
   b. DLI for patients with AML and ALL reported with 10–40% overall survival, usually limited by resistant relapse
   c. Dose determination is often based on the number of CD3+ T cells/kg recipient body weight, commonly ranging from 1×10^7 to $2\text{--}3 \times 10^8$/kg, based on the recipient's disease
   d. Determination of need for growth factor-mobilized DLI vs unstimulated DLI is influenced by the need for salvage chemotherapy
6. Second transplant
   a. Myeloablative allogeneic

      i. Success is limited by significant increases in treatment-related morbidity and mortality
- b. Reduced-intensity allogeneic
  - i. Most common consideration after failed autologous transplantation
  - ii. Clinical trials to assess coordinated tandem approach of reduced-intensity allogeneic after autologous transplantation are ongoing
7. Disease-specific chemotherapy and/or radiation
8. Biological and targeted agents
9. Supportive and palliative care

24.3 DISEASE-SPECIFIC TREATMENT FOR RELAPSE

1. AML
   - a. Withdrawal of immune suppression to stimulate a graft-vs-leukemia (GvL) effect
   - b. Re-induction chemotherapy
     - i. Idarubicin/Cytarabine (3+7)
     - ii. FLAG/Ida
     - iii. Gemtuzumab (Mylotarg®) has been used at low dose for focused treatment of the relapsed myeloid compartment with sparing of the donor CD3+ T-cell population
       - Due to toxicity and limited efficacy, FDA has recently (June, 2010) limited use of this agent to centers with active INDs
   - c. DLI
     - i. Limited response documented by clinical trials
     - ii. Toxicities include GvHD, aplasia, infections
     - iii. Most effective in slowly progressing disease
     - iv. Patients receiving DLI in CR or with MRD have better outcomes than those with higher tumor burdens
   - d. Second allogeneic transplant although many issues remain unclear
     - i. same or different donor?
     - ii. impact of timing of relapse?
     - iii. reduced-intensity vs myeloablative conditioning regimen?
   - e. Biologic and targeted therapies
     - i. Sorafenib for FLT3+ disease
     - ii. 5-azacitidine (Vidaza®) for patients with MDS has been used with success in some centers

2. ALL
   a. Withdrawal of immune suppression to induce GvL
   b. Conventional chemotherapy
      i. Hyper-CVAD
      ii. HAM
      iii. FLAG/Ida
      iv. Mito/VP-16
      v. Nelarabine (T-cell disease)
   c. Patients typically demonstrate limited survival after post-transplant relapse
   d. DLI can be considered; however, limited efficacy has been demonstrated
   e. Response rates estimated at 0–20% with few long-term survivors
3. CML
   a. The most favorable results with DLI have been documented in patients in patients with post-transplant relapse with durable remissions reaching 80%
   b. The advent of tyrosine kinase inhibitors (imatinib, dasatinib, nilotinib) has improved response rates of patients with cytogenetic relapse
   c. Convention chemotherapy may be required for patients who relapse in blast crisis
      i. Myeloid blast crisis
         – Idarubicin/cytarabine (3+7)
         – FLAG/Ida
      ii. Lymphoid blast crisis
         – HyperCVAD
         – HAM
         – FLAG/Ida
         – Mito/VP16
4. MM
   a. Relapse post-autologous transplant is anticipated as allogeneic transplant offers the only curative option at this time
   b. Depending on time from transplant to relapse, a second autologous transplant is often considered
      i. Second autologous transplant are considered to be of little benefit to patients who relapse within 1 year of their initial transplant
   c. Consideration may be given to reduced-intensity allogeneic transplant at the expense of greater morbidity and mortality from regimen-related toxicity.

d. Newer biologic agents such as lenalidomide have changed the expected clinical course of multiple myeloma, and may provide additional benefit for patients who relapse after autologous transplant

5. NHL
   a. Reduced-intensity allogeneic transplant for post-autologous transplant relapse can be efficacious; however, 2 year PFS has been reported at $\leq 35\%$
   b. Consider second autologous transplants in patients who relapse >1 year after an initial autologous transplant and have chemosensitive disease

24.4 FUTURE RESEARCH INITIATIVES

1. Exploration of mechanisms of disease resistance
   a. Generation of animal models that allow the exploration of the etiology of therapeutic resistance
   b. Novel therapeutics that target resistant disease
   c. Reduce resistance incidence with novel combination conditioning regimens or maintenance therapy
   d. Alter the rate of somatic evolution to assist in the prevention of relapse

2. Elucidation of the pathophysiology of GvL
   a. Identify maneuvers to maximally deliver GvL and promote immune reconstitution from donor T-cells with clinically insignificant GvHD
   b. Determination of new target antigens to drive immune responses, as well as to harness effector cells necessary for disease-specific responses
   c. Determine the pathways for induction, expansion, and trafficking of immune effectors that selectively recognize host hematopoietic tissues, but not the target tissues of GvHD
   d. Exploitation of novel immune suppressive regimens

3. Standardized assessment of molecular markers for hematologic malignancies
   a. Determination of the optimal timing for monitoring minimal residual disease (MRD) and chimerism after allogeneic HSCT
   b. Define the timeline for kinetic change in MRD and establishment of chimerism after allogeneic HSCT
   c. Establish strict criteria for remission and relapse that incorporate measurement of the molecular markers of hematologic malignancy

    d. Investigate novel interventional strategies utilizing changes in MRD and/or chimerism to prevent the emergence of clinical relapse

References

Bishop, R., Alyea, E., Cairo, M., Falkenburg, J., June, C., Kroger, N., et al. (2010). Introduction to the reports from the National Cancer Institute First International Workshop on the biology, prevention, and treatment of relapse after allogeneic hematopoietic stem cell transplantation. *Biol Blood Marrow Transplant*, 16:563–564.

Burzynski, J., Toro, J., Patel, R., Lee, S., Greene, R., Ochoa-Bayona, J., et al. (2009). Toxicity of a second autologous peripheral blood stem cell transplant in patients with relapsed or recurrent multiple myeloma. *Leuk Lymphoma*, 50:1442–1447.

Cairo, M., Jordan, C., Maley, C., Chao, C., Melnick, A., Armstrong, S., et al. (2010). NCI first international workshop on the biology, prevention, and treatment of relapse after allogeneic hematopoietic stem cell transplantation: Report from the committee on the biological considerations of hematological relapse following allogeneic stem cell transplantation unrelated to graft-versus-tumor effects: State of the science. *Biol Blood Marrow Tranplant*, 16: 709–728.

Devetten, M., Hari, P., Carreras, J., Logan, B., van Besien, K., Bredeson, C., et al. (2009). Unrelated donor reduced-intensity allogeneic hematopoietic stem cell transplantation for relasped and refractory Hodgkin lymphoma. *Biol Blood Marrow Transplant*, 15:109–117.

Freytes, C., Lazarus, H. (2009). Second hematopoietic SCT for lymphoma patients who relapse after autotransplantation: Another autograft or switch to allograft? *Bone Marrow Transplant*, 44: 559–569.

Kroger, N., Bacher, U., Bader, P., Bottcher, S., Borowitz, M.J., Dreger, P., et al. (2010). NCI first international workshop on the biology, prevention and treatment of relapse after allogeneic hematopoietic stem cell transplantation: Report from the committee on disease-specific methods and strategies for monitoring relapse following allogeneic stem cell transplantation. Part I: Methods, acute leukemias and myelodyspastic syndromes. *Biol Blood Marrow Transplant*, 16:1325–1346.

Miller, J., Warren, E., van den Brink, M., Ritz, J., Shlomchik, W., Murphy, W., et al. (2010). NCI first international workshop on the biology, prevention and treatment of relapse after allogeneic hematopoietic stem cell transplantation: Report from the committee on the biology underlying recurrence of malignant disease following allogeneic HSCT: Graft-versus-tumor/leukemia reaction. *Biol Blood Marrow Transplant*, 16:565–586.

Olin, R., Vogl, D., Porter, D., Luger, S., Schuster, S., Tsai, D., et al. (2009). Second auto-SCT is safe and effective salvage therapy for relapsed multiple myeloma. *Bone Marrow Transplant*, 43:417–422.

CHAPTER 25
Palliative Care

Mary Denise Smith and Amy Guthrie

There is limited research and few published articles that explore the provision of palliative care to patients and families undergoing evaluation for or receiving high-dose chemotherapy and hematopoietic stem cell transplant (HSCT). Frequently, palliative care is mistakenly seen as the consult of last resort, synonymous with hospice care, and at times a sign of failure. Patients being evaluated for or receiving disease-altering therapies may experience significant whole person suffering – pain and other physical symptoms, psychological, emotional, social and spiritual distress, uncertainty and complex decision-making. Palliative care services can be effective in responding to their experience of their illness as they continue to receive curative or disease-altering therapies until the decision is made that these therapies are no longer beneficial by either the patient or the practitioner.

25.1 DEFINITION OF PALLIATIVE MEDICINE

Palliative care is a medical subspecialty and a nursing specialty that has grown in awareness and utilization within the United States for the past two decades. Initially, this growth was in response to studies which showed that patients were not dying well as perceived by surviving family members and health care professionals. A widespread national effort was initiated to improve the care of the dying patient in the late 1990s. With further development, palliative care is now seen as a resource to assist patients to live well with advanced illness and assist with the transition to hospice when patients

R.T. Maziarz, S. Slater (eds.), *Blood and Marrow Transplant Handbook*, DOI 10.1007/978-1-4419-7506-5_25, © Springer Science+Business Media, LLC 2011

meet eligibility requirements. It is important to keep in mind that even though hospice care is always palliative care, palliative care is not always hospice care. Palliative care may be provided simultaneously with aggressive curative or disease-altering therapy and continued if the patient enrolls into a hospice program.

In 2002, the World Health Organization (WHO) revised their definition of palliative care to reflect this change. The current WHO definition for palliative care is "an approach to care which improves the quality of life for patients and families facing life threatening illnesses through the prevention, assessment and treatment of pain and other physical, psychological and spiritual problems". This specialized care is provided through an interprofessional team, which consists of a physician and an advance practice nurse at a minimum.

25.2 CORE FUNCTIONS OF PALLIATIVE CARE RELATED TO DIRECT PATIENT CARE

The skill and knowledge required to provide expert palliative care is determined by the following core functions:

1. Prevention, assessment, and treatment of pain and other physical symptoms including dyspnea, nausea, insomnia, delirium, agitation, confusion, anorexia, vomiting, constipation, and fatigue
2. Emotional, spiritual, and psychological support for patient and family
3. Communication of the expected illness trajectory while assisting the patient, or family, to clarify values and goals of care that support emotional well-being throughout the course of the disease
4. Development of a safe plan for living, connecting the patient and family with community resources that can provide adequate support
5. Transition to hospice services when the patient is eligible for assistance with terminal care

The goal for palliative care, when these functions are competently fulfilled, is that the patient and family will live well with their disease and the interventions given for disease control, and die well when further disease-altering therapies are no longer available, or the patient determines the burdens of therapies now outweigh the benefits interfering with emotional and physical well-being.

Most likely, as providers review these core functions, they say to themselves, "I do those things," and they are right. Primary palliative care is a competency that all health care professionals should demonstrate in patient care. Practitioners who provide HSCT services are challenged to alleviate the multifactoral suffering patients experience including pain, mucositis, anorexia, GvHD, diarrhea, fatigue, requirements for blood transfusion, psychological burden of disease and its treatments, and multiple problems associated with social resources or their loss. As with other aspects of practice, there are patients who require a high level of expertise in other areas – infectious diseases, cardiology, pulmonology – and referrals are made to those specialists. This same pattern is seen with referrals to palliative care specialists.

25.3 WHEN TO REFER

A referral to palliative care is indicated when the patient's needs exceed the available resources that the HSCT team can provide to address core functions of palliative care. Providers can expect the palliative care specialists to work with the HSCT team to develop a treatment plan that lessens patient and family suffering throughout the span of the curative and disease-altering therapy. Ideally, the involvement of palliative care specialists upon diagnosis, as illustrated in Fig. 25.1, can result in a greater chance of patient adherence to a treatment plan that is often described as physically and emotionally overwhelming. As disease-focused treatment continues with time, symptoms intensify and diminish. Eventually, the disease goes into remission or, alternatively, it no longer responds to disease-focused treatment. Upon achieving remission, the palliative care team can help with the patient's transition back to a life not defined by illness and treatment appointments. If the disease becomes refractory to treatment, the palliative care team can provide a seamless transition to hospice resources in the community to support the patient and family's physical, psychosocial, and spiritual needs. This transition communicates to the patient and family, "there is yet something else we can do for you", which alleviates the patient's fear of abandonment which may be magnified in the HSCT patient, when aggressive interventions are discontinued and a patient transitions to comfort care, often at alternative sites than the transplant facility.

Quality of Life Continuum for Chronic, Serious & Advanced Disease
Add Palliative Care Specialists upon diagnosis

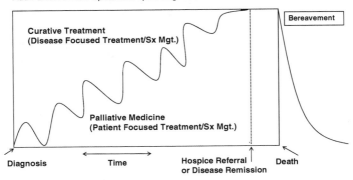

FIG. 25.1. When to add palliative care specialists to the treatment team. Quality of life continuum for chronic, serious, and advanced disease add palliative care specialists upon diagnosis

References

Chung, H., Lychkholm, L., Smith, T. (2009). Palliative care in BMT. *Bone Marrow Transplant*, 43:265–273.

Ferrel, B., Coyle, N. (2010). *Textbook of Palliative Nursing.* Oxford University Press, Cary, NC.

World Health Organization. (2001). *National Cancer Control Programmes: Policies and Managerial Guidelines.* World Health Organization, Geneva.

CHAPTER 26
Survivorship

Lisa Hansen and Brandon Hayes-Lattin

The field of cancer survivorship has matured over the past 10 years, with research efforts coordinated by transplant societies, the National Cancer Institute's Office of Cancer Survivorship, and patient advocate groups including the Lance Armstrong Foundation (http://www.livestrong.org). Most of these efforts have defined a cancer survivor as anyone living after a diagnosis of cancer, but the recommendations that follow will be directed at those survivors alive more than 1 year after transplantation.

Hematopoietic stem cell transplant (HSCT) survivors are faced with a significantly increased risk for chronic health conditions and premature death, even 10–15 years from their transplant procedure. The Bone Marrow Transplant Survivor Study (BMTSS) followed patients who survived at least 2 years post-transplant and showed that the conditional survival probability at 15 years from allogeneic transplant was 80%, with mortality rates remaining twice that of the general population after 15 years. For recipients of autologous transplant, the excess in mortality rate is also elevated for the first 10 years of survivorship before then approaching that of the general population. Careful health surveillance, healthy lifestyle choices, and prompt management of medical conditions are essential to reduce nonrelapse mortality and improve quality of life. The Center for International Blood and Marrow Transplant Research (CIBMTR) has published guidelines for patients and physicians on recommended examinations and testing for patients who have undergone both allogeneic and autologous transplantation (see Table 26.1). *Refer also to previous chapters*

R.T. Maziarz, S. Slater (eds.), *Blood and Marrow Transplant Handbook*, DOI 10.1007/978-1-4419-7506-5_26, © Springer Science+Business Media, LLC 2011

TABLE 26.1. Recommended screening and preventive practices for post-transplant patients

Recommended screening and prevention	6 Months	1 Year	Annually
Liver			
Liver function testing	All	All	As indic.
Serum ferritin		All	As indic.
Respiratory			
Clinical pulmonary assessment	All	All	All
Smoking tobacco avoidance	All	All	All
Pulmonary function testing		Allo only	As indic.
Chest radiography	As. Indic.	As indic.	As indic.
Musculoskeletal			
Bone density testing (women and patients with prolonged corticosteroid or calcineurin inhibitor use)		All	As indic.
Screen for corticosteroid-induced muscle weakness	cGvHD	cGvHD	cGvHD
Consider need for physical therapy consultation	cGvHD	cGvHD	cGvHD
Osteopenia prophylaxis with bisphosphonates recommended by some experts		cGvHD	cGvHD
Kidney			
Blood pressure screening	All	All	All
Urine protein screening	All	All	As indic.
BUN/creatinine testing	All	All	All
Nervous system			
Neurological clinical evaluation		All	As indic.

TABLE 26.1. (Continued)

Recommended screening and prevention	6 Months	1 Year	Annually
Endocrine			
Thyroid function testing		All	As indic.
Growth velocity in children		All	All
Gonadal function assessment (prepubertal boys and girls)	All	All	All
Gonadal function assessment (postpubertal women)		All	All
Vascular			
Cardiovascular risk factor assessment		All	All
Immune system			
Encapsulated organism prophylaxis	cGvHD	cGvHD	cGvHD
PCP prophylaxis	All	cGvHD	cGvHD
CMV testing	cGvHD	cGvHD	
Antifungal prophylaxis is recommended by some experts	cGvHD	cGvHD	cGvHD
Prophylaxis for HSV is recommended by some experts	cGvHD	cGvHD	cGvHD
Endocarditis prophylaxis with dental procedures–AHA guidelines		Allo only	Allo only
Immunizations – see Chapter 13	All	All	All

TABLE 26.1. (*Continued*)

Recommended screening and prevention	6 Months	1 Year	Annually
Second cancers			
Second cancer vigilance counseling		All	All
Breast/skin/testes self-exam		All	All
Clinical screening for second cancers		All	All
Pap smear/mammogram (over age 40)		All	All
Psychosocial			
Psychosocial/QOL clinical assessment	All	All	All
Mental health counseling for recognized psychosocial problems	As indic.	As indic.	As indic.
Sexual function assessment	All	All	All
Oral complications			
Dental assessment	All	All	All
Ocular			
Ocular clinical symptom evaluation	All	All	All
Schirmer testing		cGvHD	cGvHD
Ocular fundus exam		All	As indic.

All = Allogeneic and autologous patients. cGvHD = Recommended for any patient with ongoing chronic GVHD or immunosuppression

As indic. = Reassessment recommended for abnormal testing in a previous time period or for new signs/symptoms

Source: Adapted from Rizzo, J.D., Wingard, J.R., Tichelli, A., et al. (2006). Recommended screening and preventive practices for long-term survivors after hematopoietic cell transplantation: joint recommendations of the European Group for Blood and Marrow Transplantation, Center for International Blood and Marrow Transplant Research, and the American Society for Blood and Marrow Transplantation. *Biol Blood Marrow Transplant*, 12:138–151

that address specific organ systems, infection prophylaxis, and chronic graft-versus-host disease.

26.1 INFECTION

The risk of serious infection persists in HSCT patients months to years after their transplant procedure. Laboratory evidence of immune recovery generally occurs at 12 months for autologous patients, but may be delayed beyond 18 months in allogeneic recipients. Chapters 8 and 14, along with published guidelines (see Tomblyn et al.), provide recommendations for infection prophylaxis.

1. Risk factors for late infection
   a. Presence of chronic GvHD
   b. Ongoing immunosuppressive therapy
   c. HLA-mismatched or T-cell-depleted graft
   d. Presence of disease relapse
2. Surveillance
   a. CBC
   b. Immune reconstitution assessment
      i. BMT CTN recommendations
         – CD3, CD4, CD8, CD45RA/R0, CD56, CD16, CD19, and CD20 at 2, 4, 6, 12, 18, 24, and 36 months post-allogeneic transplant
         – PHA and MLC at 6, 12, 19, 24, and 36 months post-allogeneic transplant
         – NK cell function at 1, 3, 6, and 12 months post-allogeneic transplant
         – Quantitative immunoglobulins at 2, 6, 12, 18, 24, and 36 months post-allogeneic transplant
   c. CMV antigen or CMV PCR for allogeneic recipients as indicated
3. Interventions
   a. After 1 year, infection prophylaxis is individualized based on immune reconstitution (see Chapter 14)
   b. Antimicrobial prophylaxis for encapsulated bacteria, pneumocystis, and yeast/mold
   c. Post-transplant vaccinations based on published guidelines (see Chapter 13)

26.2 CARDIOVASCULAR

HSCT survivors are twice as likely to die from cardiac conditions as the general population. Reduced carotid artery distensibility has been demonstrated in a cohort of pediatric HSCT survivors. Precocious coronary arteriosclerosis develops when the heart is encompassed in the radiation field.

1. Risk factors
   a. Prior anthracycline chemotherapy (doses of >250/m^2 in autologous patients increased risk of CHF 30-fold)
   b. Radiation therapy: Thoracic radiotherapy with heart in radiation field, total body radiation
   c. Metabolic syndrome (increased blood pressure, elevated insulin levels, excess body fat, abnormal cholesterol levels)
   d. Family history of cardiovascular disease
2. Surveillance
   a. Blood pressure monitoring
   b. Serum cholesterol and blood lipids
   c. ECG and/or echocardiogram as clinically indicated
3. Interventions
   a. Reduce or eliminate modifiable risk factors (maintain optimal blood pressure and body weight, cholesterol and blood lipid management, smoking cessation)
   b. Cardiology referral and evaluation as indicated

26.3 PULMONARY

Serious pulmonary complications generally develop during the first weeks or months post-HSCT. However, pulmonary function can become compromised in long-term survivors as a consequence of late infection, obstructive or restrictive disease.

1. Risk factors
   a. Chronic GvHD
   b. Immunosuppressive medications
   c. CMV disease
   d. Busulfan or total body radiation conditioning
   e. Pre-transplant pulmonary function abnormalities
   f. Older age
2. Surveillance
   a. Pulse oximetry
   b. Pulmonary function testing (PFT) for allogeneic recipients at 1 year; however, as early presentation of bronchiolitis obliterans is asymptomatic and prognosis is poor for symptomatic disease, consideration should be made to begin PFT monitoring as early as 3 months post-transplant.

c. Closer PFT monitoring (every 3–6 months) may be indicated in patients with cGvHD
d. Appropriate imaging for symptomatic patients (CXR, CT scan)

3. Prevention and interventions
See Chapter 19 for management of pulmonary complications.
a. Annual influenza vaccination for patients and household contacts
b. Smoking cessation
c. Education of patient and family on infection control measures to reduce exposure to community respiratory viral infections
d. Prompt treatment of respiratory infections

26.4 NEUROLOGIC

1. Cognitive dysfunction
Pediatric HSCT survivors suffer the greatest burden of neurologic effects post-transplant. Adult HSCT patients can be plagued by cognitive dysfunction, but most recover normal function by 1 year.
a. Risk factors
    i. Patient age
    ii. Unrelated donor allogeneic > matched sibling allogeneic > autologous
    iii. Prior cranial radiation or intrathecal therapy
    iv. Possible genetic predisposition – E4 allele of apolipoprotein
    v. Preexisting cognitive deficits
b. Surveillance and diagnosis
    i. Neurologic exam
        – Careful history from patient and family of intellectual, social, and physical functioning
    ii. Serum electrolytes, LFTs, serum creatinine
    iii. MRI of brain if indicated
    iv. Referral for neurologic consultation and neuropsychological testing as indicated
c. Interventions
    i. Treatment is individualized, based on age, degree of cognitive disruption, and presumed etiology
    ii. Research suggests physical exercise improves cognitive function

2. Peripheral neuropathy

Ten to twenty percent of patients treated for malignant disease have peripheral neuropathy. This impairs mobility, increases fall risk, and may require chronic narcotic analgesia. Neuropathy symptoms can gradually improve over time.

   a. Risk factors
      i. History of treatment with neurotoxic chemotherapeutic agents (vinca alkyloids, platinum compounds, bortezimib, thalidomide, taxanes)
      ii. Calcineurin inhibitors
      iii. Older age
      iv. Diabetes mellitus and liver disease can exacerbate preexisting symptoms

   b. Interventions
      i. Gamma aminobutyric acid for painful neuropathy
         – Gabapentin (Neurontin®) beginning at 100–300 mg po qhs, increasing dose to 900–3600 mg daily in dose increments of 50–100% every 3 days. Slower titration recommended for elderly or medically frail patients. Dose adjust for renal insufficiency.
         – Pregabalin (Lyrica®) 50 mg po TID, may be increased to 100 mg po TID. Slower titration recommended for elderly or medically frail patients. Dose adjust for renal insufficiency.
      ii. Antidepressants (e.g., duloxetine [Cymbalta®] 30–60 mg po daily, titrated up to 60–120 mg po daily) for burning pain
      iii. Narcotic analgesics
      iv. Consider available clinical trials

26.5 ENDOCRINE

1. Hypothyroidism

Hypothyroidism is a common late complication of HSCT, developing in 15–25% of patients.

   a. Risk factors
      i. Total body irradiation
      ii. Involved field radiotherapy to the neck region
      iii. High-dose alkylating agents in conditioning regimen (busulfan, cyclophosphamide)

   b. Surveillance

    i. Annual thyroid function testing, particularly patients treated with TBI

  c. Interventions

    i. Thyroid hormone replacement

    ii. Monitoring thyroid function tests at 6 weeks post-therapy, then every 6 months

2. Diabetes

Steroid-induced diabetes is common in allogeneic transplant patients requiring long-term corticosteroids for control of cGvHD. Metabolic syndrome (abdominal obesity, dyslipidemia, hyperglycemia, and hypertension) predisposes patients to type 2 diabetes and cardiovascular disease. Findings from the Bone Marrow Transplant Survivors Study (BMTSS) revealed that allogeneic HSCT recipients were 3.7 times more likely to report a diagnosis of diabetes than their matched sibling cohort. Obesity and at least two components of metabolic syndrome were increased nearly threefold in childhood cancer survivors.

  a. Risk factors

    i. Corticosteroid therapy

    ii. Obesity

    iii. Family history

    iv. Physical inactivity

  b. Surveillance

    i. Annual fasting blood glucose, Hgb A1C, lipid panel for patients at risk.

  c. Interventions

    i. Hypoglycemic agents, dietary modification, exercise program

    ii. Close monitoring for cardiovascular risk factors

26.6 MUSCULOSKELETAL COMPLICATIONS

1. Osteoporosis may develop prematurely secondary to chronic corticosteroids or medical menopause in women (see Chapter 13 for further recommendations)

  a. Surveillance

    i. Patients should be counseled regarding their risk for osteoporosis

    ii. Bone densitometry scan at 1 year post-transplant, then yearly depending on severity of osteopenia/osteoporosis

  b. Interventions

      i. Oral or intravenous bisphosphonates
      ii. Calcium and vitamin D supplementation
      iii. Regular weight-bearing exercise as tolerated
      iv. Consider estrogen replacement for women (evaluate risk-benefit)

2. Avascular necrosis

Avascular necrosis (AVN) is a late complication with a reported incidence of 4–10%. AVN tends to affect weight-bearing joints in a bilateral distribution. Hips are most commonly affected. Knees, ankles, and wrists can also develop AVN.

   a. Risk factors
      i. Long-term corticosteroid therapy
      ii. Total body radiation, particularly high total doses
   b. Surveillance and diagnosis
      i. Routine surveillance is not indicated
      ii. Careful patient history, focusing on joint pain quality, intensity, and duration
      iii. MRI of symptomatic joints
   c. Interventions/analgesics
   d. Orthopedic devices
   e. Definitive treatment necessitates total joint replacement

26.7 SECONDARY MALIGNANT NEOPLASMS (SMNs)

Individuals diagnosed with a malignancy are twice as likely to develop a second cancer as individuals, matched by age and gender, who lack a cancer history. For HSCT survivors, the risk is magnified two to three times. The incidence of SMNs in HSCT survivors increases over time and varies among different studies (from 3 to >10%).

1. Risk factors
   a. Diagnosis of Hodgkin's lymphoma
   b. Preparative regimens containing total body radiation
   c. ATG-containing preparative regimens
   d. Long-term immunosuppressive therapy
   e. Chronic GvHD
2. SMNs in HSCT survivors
   a. Basal and squamous cell carcinomas of the skin
   b. Squamous cell carcinoma of the oral cavity
   c. Other solid tumors: liver, cervix, thyroid, bone/connective tissue

    d. CNS tumors

    e. Non-Hodgkin's lymphomas

    f. MDS/AML

    g. Post-transplant lymphoproliferative disorder (PTLD)

3. Surveillance

    a. Survivor counseling regarding increased risk, self-monitoring for signs and symptoms

    b. Physical exam with specific attention to signs and symptoms of SMNs

    c. Dermatology referral as indicated

    d. CBC, comprehensive chemistry panel

    e. Routine cancer screening tests (mammography, Pap smear, colonoscopy, etc).

4. Counseling and interventions

    a. Lifestyle modifications to reduce risk: smoking avoidance, healthy diet, exercise to maintain normal weight

    b. Sunscreen and sun-protective clothing

    c. PTLD may be effectively managed with a reduction in immunosuppressive medications and administration of anti-B cell monoclonal antibody therapy (e.g., rituximab)

5. Outcome of secondary MDS/AML is generally poor despite aggressive therapy

26.8 SEXUALITY AND REPRODUCTIVE ISSUES

1. Infertility

Gonadal dysfunction and infertility is prevalent and distressing for young adults who have undergone HSCT. Medical advances such as in vitro fertilization, improved infertility drug regimens, pretreatment sperm donation and ovary harvest/storage, egg donation, and other high technology approaches make pregnancy feasible for increasing numbers of cancer survivors.

    a. Risk factors

        i. Age >30

        ii. Female sex

        iii. Total body radiation

        iv. Alkylating agents

    b. Diagnosis

        i. Females

            – Amenorrhea

- FSH in menopausal range on two consecutive tests, at least 1 month apart
- Low estradiol levels
  ii. Males
  - Elevated FSH
  - azoospermia
  c. Interventions and education
   i. Ideally, fertility issues and methods for preserving fertility are addressed at diagnosis prior to initiation of chemotherapy and/or radiation
   ii. Referral to a reproductive endocrinologist for sperm or embryo cryopreservation
   iii. Counseling regarding parenthood options including fertilization maneuvers, surrogacy, and adoption
   iv. Observational studies suggest high-dose therapy does not increase risk of congenital abnormalities or cancer in offspring
   v. Evidence lacking on safe interval from HSCT to conception. In general, females should allow 6 months before conception; males possibly 2 years
   vi. Female patients receiving total body radiation are at increased risk of miscarriage, premature birth, and neonatal low birth weight
2. Sexual dysfunction
  A recent longitudinal study revealed that nearly 50% of men and 80% of women have long-term sexual problems after HSCT. While most males recover to pre-HSCT function, most females do not. Both male and female survivors report inferior sexual function when compared with healthy controls, even 5 years from HSCT. Sexual activity and satisfaction are both adversely affected.
  a. Possible mechanisms
   i. Females
   - pituitary axis damage from alkylating agents, total body radiation
   - ovarian failure
   - radiation-induced vaginal stenosis
   - vaginal mucosal changes associated with GvHD
   - depression and other psychosocial factors
   ii. Males
   - pituitary axis damage from alkylating agents, total body radiation
   - testicular insufficiency
   - cavernosal arterial insufficiency

- hypothyroidism
- depression and other psychosocial factors
b. Evaluation and interventions
    i. Encouraging discussion of sexual concerns
    ii. Females
        - thyroid function tests; FSH and estradiol
        - instruct patient and provide vaginal lubricants, dilator or vibrator
        - consider estrogen replacement therapy (weigh risk/benefit); testosterone
        - referral to gynecologist and/or sexual therapist.
    iii. Males
        - thyroid function tests; testosterone level (usually returns to normal by 2 years post-ASCT)
        - trial of phosphodiesterase 5 inhibitor if not contraindicated
            • sildenafil citrate (Viagra®) 25–100 mg po 1 h prior to sexual activity
            • tadalafil (Cialis®) 2.5 mg po daily, may increase to 5 mg po daily as tolerated; or for intermittent use, 10 mg po prior to sexual activity may increase or 20 mg po prior to sexual activity as tolerated.
        - referral to urologist and/or sexual therapist.

26.9 PSYCHOSOCIAL CONCERNS

Depression, anxiety, and post-traumatic stress disorder (PTSD) compound the physical challenges associated with long-term recovery from HSCT. Astute clinicians will include a careful history to screen for depression and psychosocial adjustment disorders during follow-up visits. Formal quality of life (QOL) studies indicate that autologous transplant patients enjoy excellent QOL at 1 year post-transplant. Allogeneic survivors report good to excellent QOL at 1 year, but the presence of cGvHD negatively affects physical functioning scores in most patients

TABLE 26.1. Resource lists are available to survivors and their caregivers at the following web sites:

NCI Office of Cancer Survivorship	http://cancercontrol.cancer.gov/ocs/
Lance Armstrong Foundation	http://www.livestrong.org
National Marrow Donor Program	http:///www.marrow.org
National Bone Marrow Transplant Link	http://www.nbmtlink.org

at 1 year. Persistent concerns include physical functioning, sexual satisfaction, difficulties with health and life insurance, and returning to work or school.

References

Armenian, S.H., Sun, C.L., Francisco, L., Steinberger, J., Kurian, S., Wong, F.L., et al. (2008). Late congestive heart failure after hematopoietic cell transplantation. *J Clin Oncol*, 26:5537–5543.

Bahtia, S., Francisco, L., Carter, A., Sun, C.L., Baker, K.S., Gurney, J.G., et al. (2007). Late mortality after allogeneic hematopoietic cell transplantation and functional status of long term survivors: Report from the bone marrow transplant survivor study. *Blood*, 110:3784–3792.

Bahtia, S., Robinson, L.L., Francisco, L., Carter, A., Liu, Y., Grant, M., et al. (2005). Late mortality in survivors of autologous hematopoietic cell transplantation: Report from the bone marrow transplant survivor study. *Blood*, 110:4215–4222.

Baker, K.S., Armenian, S., Bhatia, S. (2010). Long-term consequences of hematopoietic stem cell transplantation: Current state of the science. *Biol Blood Marrow Transplant*, 16:S90–S96.

Carter, A., Robison, L.L., Francisco, L., Smith, D., Grant, M., Baker, K.S., et al. (2006). Prevalence of conception and pregnancy outcomes after hematopoietic cell transplantation: Report from the bone marrow transplant survivor study. *Bone Marrow Transplant*, 37:1023–1029.

Campbell, J., Moravec, C.K. (2004). Long-term complications of hematopoietic stem cell transplantation. In P.C. Buchsel P.M. Kapustay (Eds.), *Stem Cell Transplantation: A Clinical Textbook* (pp. 23.3–23.16).Oncology Nursing Society, Pittsburgh, PA.

Chao, N.J., Tierney, D.K., Bloom, J.R., Long, G.D., Barr, T.A., Stallbaum, B.A., et al. (1992). Dynamic assessment of quality of life after autologous bone marrow transplantation. *Blood*, 80:825–830.

Chiodi, S., Spinelli, S., Ravera, G., Petti, A.R., Van Lint M.T., Lamparelli, T., et al. (2000). Quality of life in 244 recipients of allogeneic bone marrow transplantation. *Br J Haematol*, 110:614–619.

Flowers, M.E.D. Deeg, J.H. (2003). Delayed complications after hematopoietic cell transplantation. In K.G. Blume, S.J. Forman, F.R. Appelbaum (Eds.), *Thomas' Hematopoietic Cell Transplantation* (3rd ed., pp. 944–961).Blackwell Science, Malden, MA.

Hertnestein, B., Stefanic, M., Schmeiser, T., Scholz, M., Göller, V., Clausen, M., et al. (1994). Cardiac toxicity of bone marrow transplantation: Predictive value of cardiologic evaluation before transplant. *J Clin Oncol*, 12:998–1004.

Kalaycio, M., Pohlman, B., Kuczkowski, E., Rybicki, L., Andresen, S., Sobecks, R., et al. (2006). High-dose busulfan and the risk of pulmonary mortality after autologous stem cell transplant. *Clin Transplant*, 20:783–787.

Kolb, H.J., Socie, G., Duell, T., Van Lint, M.T., Tichelli, A., Apperley, J.F., et al. (1999). Malignant neoplasms in long-term survivors of bone marrow transplantation. Late effects working party of the European cooperative group for blood and Marrow transplantation and the European late effect project group. *Ann Intern Med*, 131:738–744.

Myers, J.S. (2009). Chemotherapy-related cognitive impairment: Neuroimaging, neuropsychiatric testing and the neuropsychologist. *Clin J Oncol Nurs*, 13:413–421.

Rizzo, J.D., Wingard, J.R., Tichelli, A., Lee, S.J., Van Lint, M.T., Burns, L.J., et al. (2006). Recommended screening and preventive practices for long-term survivors after hematopoietic cell transplantation: Joint recommendations of the European group for Blood and Marrow Transplantation, Center for International Blood and Marrow Transplant Research, and the American Society for Blood and Marrow Transplantation. *Biol Blood Marrow Transplant*, 12:138–151.

Rizzo, J.D., Curtis, R.E., Socie, G., Sobocinski, K.A., Gilbert, E., Landgren, O., et al. (2009). Solid cancers after allogeneic hematopoietic cell transplantation. *Blood*, 113:1175–1183.

Syralia, K.L., Kurland, B.F., Abrams, J.R., Sanders, J.E., Heiman, J.R. (2008). Sexual function changes during the 5 years after high-dose treatment and hematopoietic cell transplantation for malignancy, with case-matched controls at 5 years. *Blood*, 111:989–996.

Tomblyn M., Chiller, T., Einsele, H. Gress, R., Sepkowitz, K., Storek, J., et al. (2009). Guidelines for preventing infectious complications among hematopoietic cell transplant recipients: A global perspective. *Biol Blood Marrow Transplant*, 15:1143–1238.

Wickham, R. (2007). Chemotherapy-induced peripheral neuropathy: A review and implications for oncology nursing practice. *Clin J Oncol Nurs*, 11:361–376.

Appendices

APPENDIX 1: PROCEDURE – BONE MARROW ASPIRATE AND BIOPSY

Indication: Evaluate marrow for disease involvement; restaging; evaluate cytopenias.

Procedure:

1. Contact the Bone Marrow Bench to schedule a technician for the procedure.
2. Complete all appropriate requisitions or electronic orders as outlined below.
3. Identify the patient and complete TEAM PAUSE documentation.
4. Obtain written consent. If patient requests medication for anxiolysis, indicate this on the consent form and ascertain that the patient *is accompanied by a driver*.
5. Obtain a bone marrow biopsy tray. This should contain an 11 g 4″ aspirate needle and a 11 g 4″ biopsy needle, a 30 mL luer lock syringe, a 10 mL syringe with 21, 20, and 25 g needles, 10 mL lidocaine 1%, scalpel, paper drapes, Betadine swabsticks, 4×4 gauze sponges, and an adhesive bandage. Also obtain sterile gloves.
6. Position the patient in the prone position and prepare your supplies.
7. Identify the iliac crest. Prepare the biopsy site with Betadine, put on your sterile gloves and drape the area.
8. Administer local anesthesia using lidocaine 1%. Begin by forming a wheal on the skin. Continue to numb the area with lidocaine through the fatty layer down to the bone.

R.T. Maziarz, S. Slater (eds.), *Blood and Marrow Transplant Handbook*, DOI 10.1007/978-1-4419-7506-5, © Springer Science+Business Media, LLC 2011

Administer lidocaine in a widening circular area over the surface of the bone completely infiltrating the periosteum.

9. Prepare your syringes to obtain aspirate specimens. The bone marrow technician will provide additional sterile syringes and sodium heparin to use during the procedure.

10. Using the scalpel, make a single cutaneous incision to the hub of the scalpel to allow easy passage of the aspirate needle.

11. Insert the aspirate needle through the skin incision until contact with the bone is made. Using gentle, steady, rotating pressure, continue until the needle is firmly seated in the marrow space.

    a. The first aspirate should be a quick pull into an unheparinized syringe (1–2 mL). Slides should be made from this specimen if spicules are present. The remainder of the specimen should be sent for morphology.

    b. If same-sex chimerisms are required, the second specimen should be sent for VNTR in an unheparinized syringe.

    c. Specimens which should be sent in a heparinized syringe include flow cytometry, cytogenetics, and FISH studies, along with samples for appropriate research studies.

    d. Any additional specimens should be sent per lab guidelines.

    e. Please keep in mind that collection methods and sample collection varies from institution to institution. Your institution's guidelines should be followed to ensure adequate interpretation of the sample.

12. Once the aspirates have been collected, remove the aspirate needle. Insert the biopsy needle through the skin incision until contact with the bone is made. Using gentle, steady, rotating pressure, introduce the needle through the cortex slightly into the marrow space. Remove the trochar and continue to advance the needle further into the marrow space to obtain a core biopsy. Using the trochar, measure the approximate length of the core by inserting it back through the biopsy needle. Once the core measures at least 2 cm, break the core biopsy off by rotating the biopsy needle multiple times.

13. Remove the biopsy needle and attach the needle guard to the bottom of the biopsy needle. Insert the shepherd's hook through the bottom of the needle to dislodge the core

onto a sterile gauze or slide provided by the bone marrow technician.

14. Once adequate specimens have been obtained, hold pressure to the biopsy site until bleeding has stopped and apply a clean bandage.

15. Assist the patient to the supine position and observe for 10–15 min for signs of bleeding. The patient may require longer observation if anxiolysis was used.

16. Instruct the patient to keep the bandage clean and dry for 24 h. The bandage may then be removed. Also instruct the patient to call should any signs of infection develop.

17. Document the procedure in the patient's medical record.

STANDARD TESTS FOR MARROW STUDIES

1. Acute myeloid leukemia
   a. At diagnosis
      1. morphology
      2. flow cytometry
      3. cytogenetics
      4. FISH studies pending MD input e.g., t(15;17), t(9;21)
      5. FLT-3, NPM-1, c-kit
   b. Subsequent marrow studies
      1. morphology
      2. flow cytometry
      3. cytogenetics (not indicated on day 14 marrow studies)
      4. FISH for previous abnormalities, if applicable
2. Acute lymphoid leukemia
   a. At diagnosis
      1. morphology
      2. flow cytometry
      3. cytogenetics
      4. FISH for BCR/abl, MLL locus
   b. Subsequent marrow studies
      1. morphology
      2. flow cytometry
      3. cytogenetics (not indicated on day 14 marrow studies)
      4. FISH for previous abnormalities, if applicable
3. Chronic myeloid leukemia
   a. At diagnosis
      1. morphology

       2. flow cytometry
       3. cytogenetics
       4. FISH for BCR/abl
    b. Subsequent marrow studies
       1. Morphology
       2. flow cytometry (only required if accelerated phase or blast crisis is suspected)
       3. cytogenetics
       4. FISH for previous abnormalities, if applicable
       5. PCR for BCR/abl is *not indicated* – this is done on peripheral blood only

4. Chronic lymphoid leukemia
    a. At diagnosis
       1. morphology
       2. flow cytometry
       3. cytogenetics
       4. FISH for CLL panel (chromosome 11, 13, 17 abnormalities)
    b. Subsequent marrow studies
       1. morphology
       2. flow cytometry
       3. cytogenetics
       4. FISH for CLL panel

5. Myelodysplastic syndrome
    a. At diagnosis
       1. morphology
       2. flow cytometry
       3. cytogenetics
       4. FISH for 5q and deletion 7
    b. Subsequent marrow studies
       1. morphology
       2. flow cytometry
       3. cytogenetics
       4. FISH for previous abnormalities, if applicable

6. Myelofibrosis
    a. At diagnosis
       1. morphology
       2. flow cytometry (if AML is suspected)
       3. cytogenetics
       4. JAK-2 mutation
    b. Subsequent marrow studies
       1. morphology
       2. flow cytometry (if suspect progression to AML)

3. cytogenetics
4. FISH for previous abnormalities, if applicable
7. Non-Hodgkin's lymphoma
   a. At diagnosis
      1. morphology
      2. flow cytometry
      3. if mantle cell lymphoma, FISH for t(11;14)
      4. if follicular lymphoma, PCR for t(14;18)
   b. Subsequent marrow studies
      1. morphology
      2. flow cytometry
      3. if marrow is done to assess disease status prior to stem cell mobilization, cytogenetics are indicated
8. Hodgkin's disease
   a. At diagnosis
      1. morphology
      2. flow cytometry
   b. Subsequent marrow studies
      1. morphology
      2. flow cytometry
9. Multiple myeloma
   a. At diagnosis
      1. morphology
      2. flow cytometry
      3. cytogenetics
      4. FISH for myeloma panel [t(11;14), t(4;14), t(14;16), 17p, 13]
      5. Congo red stain to r/o amyloid
   b. Subsequent marrow studies
      1. morphology
      2. flow cytometry
      3. FISH for previous abnormalities, if applicable
10. Post-transplant marrow studies
    a. Follow above parameters for diagnosis
    b. FISH for XY for opposite sex donors or VNTR for same-sex donors to assess chimerisms

APPENDIX 2: PROCEDURE: LUMBAR PUNCTURE

Indications:

– Diagnostic: r/o CNS leukemia/lymphoma, r/o infection
– Therapeutic: instillation of intrathecal chemotherapy

Procedure:

1. Review lab studies to verify patient's platelet count is >50,000/mm^3. If platelet count is <50,000/mm^3, transfuse one single-donor irradiated platelet product and check a post-platelet count. Continue to transfuse single-donor irradiated platelet products to achieve a platelet count >50,000/mm^3.
2. If chemotherapy will be administered during the procedure, submit the orders to pharmacy for mixing. All intrathecal chemotherapy should be mixed in preservative-free normal saline only. Chemotherapy should be checked prior to administration according to institutional policy.
3. Place the orders for CSF studies in the patient's chart or electronic medical record. These typically include:
   a. tube 1 – protein, glucose.
   b. tube 2 – cell count and differential
   c. tube 3 – flow cytometry and cytology
   d. tube 4 – cultures for diagnostic studies, if indicated
4. Identify the patient and complete TEAM PAUSE documentation.
5. Obtain written consent. If patient requests medication for anxiolysis, indicate this on the consent form and ascertain that the patient *is accompanied by a driver*.
6. Obtain lumbar puncture tray. This should contain a 20 g 3$\frac{1}{2}$ needle with stylet, a 3 mL syringe with 25 g and 22 g needles, 2 mL lidocaine 1%, four numbered specimen vials, gauze pads, Betadine swabsticks, paper drapes, and an adhesive bandage. Also obtain sterile gloves.
7. Place the patient in the lateral decubitus position, curled into the fetal position and prepare your supplies.
8. Locate the sacral promontory. The end of this structure coincides with the L5-S1 interspace. Use this reference to locate the L4-L5 interspace.
8. Using sterile technique, prep the skin over L4-L5 with betadine and drape the area.
9. Administer local anesthesia using lidocaine 1%. Begin by forming a wheal on the skin. Continue to numb the deeper

tissue with lidocaine, positioning the needle toward the umbilicus.

10. Insert the spinal needle bevel up through the skin and into the deeper tissue. Aim the needle toward the umbilicus. A slight pop will be felt when the dura is punctured. If you hit bone, partially withdraw the needle, reposition, and attempt again.

11. Once inside the dura, remove the stylet. If fluid does not flow, re-insert the stylet and attempt to enter the dura again. This may require slight advancement or partial withdrawal and repositioning.

12. Once CSF flows, collect the appropriate specimens in the numbered tubes.

13. If chemotherapy is to be administered during the procedure, attach the chemotherapy syringe to the hub of the spinal needle once fluid collection is completed, keeping one hand sterile.

14. Slowly inject the chemotherapy over a period of 2 to 3 min, checking for flow every 2 to 3 mL.

15. Once fluid collection and chemotherapy administration are completed, withdraw the needle and apply gentle pressure to the insertion site. Apply a clean bandage.

16. Instruct the patient to lie flat for 1 to 4 h to avoid post-procedure headache.

17. Document the procedure in the patient's medical record.

APPENDIX 3: PROCEDURE – OMMAYA RESERVOIR TAP
Indications:

– Diagnostic: r/o CNS leukemia/lymphoma, r/o infection
– Therapeutic: instillation of intrathecal chemotherapy

Procedure:

1. If chemotherapy will be administered during the procedure, submit the orders to pharmacy for mixing. All intrathecal chemotherapy should be mixed in preservative-free normal saline only. Chemotherapy should be checked prior to administration per institutional policy.
2. Place the orders for CSF studies in the patient's chart or electronic medical record. These typically include:
   a. tube 1 – protein, glucose
   b. tube 2 – cell count and differential
   c. tube 3 – flow cytometry and cytology
   d. tube 4 – cultures for diagnostic studies, if indicated.
3. Identify the patient and complete TEAM PAUSE documentation.
4. Obtain written consent. If patient requests medication for anxiolysis, indicate this on the consent form and ascertain that the patient *is accompanied by a driver*.
5. Obtain supplies including: 10 mL luer-lock syringe, 25 g butterfly needle, Betadine swabsticks, sterile 2×2 gauze pads, and an adhesive bandage. Also obtain sterile gloves.
6. Place the patient in the supine position with the head of bed elevated approximately 30°. Locate the Ommaya reservoir and pump the port gently three times to ensure flow.
7. Using sterile technique, prep the skin over the port.
8. Insert the needle into the center of the port until the needle strikes the back of the port. Observe for flow of CSF.
9. Attach the sterile syringe to the butterfly needle and slowly withdraw 6 mL of CSF.
10. Once the specimen has been collected, attach the syringe containing chemotherapy and slowly inject the chemotherapy over a period of 2 to 3 min, checking for flow after every 2 to 3 mL.
11. Remove the needle from the Ommaya and hold gentle pressure to the site until the bleeding has stopped. Apply a clean bandage.
12. Instruct the patient to lie flat for 1 to 4 h to avoid post-procedural headache.
13. Distribute the specimen into 3 to 4 glass red-top tubes for processing in the lab.
14. Document the procedure in the patient's medical record.

APPENDIX 4: PROCEDURE: SKIN BIOPSY

Indication: Evaluation of rash or other skin lesion, r/o GvHD, infection, etc.

Procedure:

1. Identify the patient's affected areas of skin to be biopsied and mark those areas.
2. Obtain topical anesthetic, either topical anesthetic spray (e.g., Flori-Methane) or Elamax cream. If using Elamax cream, apply 2.5 g (approximately 1/2 of a 5 g tube) in a thick layer over the site to be biopsied. Cover with an occlusive dressing (Op-Site/Tegaderm). Note the time of application on the dressing. A minimum of 1 h is necessary to obtain analgesic effect. If using anesthetic spray, spray area to be biopsied for 3–5 s at a distance of approximately 12 inches. Do not frost the skin. Note: Intradermal injections of Lidocaine may distort the histologic architecture, so the use of Elamax cream or anesthetic spray is encouraged.
3. Obtain skin biopsy tray which should contain 3 or 4 mm punch biopsy needle, scalpel, scissors, forceps, needle driver, cloth/paper drapes, betadine swabsticks, alcohol wipes, 4×4 gauze sponges, 5-0 nylon suture material and a specimen container with formalin. A syringe, 1% Lidocaine, and sterile gloves should also be available. A suture removal kit may be used to obtain some of the specimens.
4. After a minimum of 1 h application of the Elamax cream, remove the occlusive dressing and wipe off the Elamax cream. Prepare and lay out required supplies. Using sterile technique, prepare the biopsy sites with Betadine, put on gloves, and apply drape if necessary. Apply anesthetic spray, if using.
5. Place the punch biopsy needle on the skin and exert moderate downward pressure. Rotate the punch biopsy needle until the entire blade is within the skin, then remove the biopsy needle.
6. Using forceps, gently pull the punch from the skin, which will leave the base of tissue attached to the subcutaneous layer of tissue. Using scissors, cut the base of the biopsy and lift it free from the surrounding tissue.
7. Place the specimen in the formalin solution and label the container with the patient's identifying data.

8. Blot or apply pressure briefly to the biopsy site with gauze, then suture or steri-strip site as needed. If the patient experiences discomfort at the biopsy site during suturing, intradermal Lidocaine should be used at this time.

9. Apply a small amount antibacterial ointment to biopsy site and cover with occlusive dressing. Instruct patient to leave dressing in place for 24 h. After 24 h, remove the dressing. Apply small amount of antibacterial ointment to biopsy site twice a day. Instruct the patient/caregiver to notify the nursing staff if redness, swelling, persistent or colored drainage, or discomfort occurs at the biopsy site.

10. Complete an appropriate requisition and send specimen to Dermatopathology per institutional guidelines.

11. Remove the sutures in 7–10 days.

12. Document the procedure in the patient's medical record.

APPENDIX 5: OHSU LOW-BACTERIA DIET

Below is the low bacteria diet currently in use at Oregon Health & Science University. It is intended to be an example of one institution's practice.

INPATIENT

Certain whole, undamaged fresh fruit and vegetables are allowed as long as they are thoroughly washed with water by a RN, CNA, or family member. (*The ones denoted with asterisks will be provided by the dietary service.)

ALLOWED ITEMS THAT MUST BE WASHED AND PEELED

*Apple melons	lime	cucumber	
*Orange	peach	pineapple	carrot
*Banana	kiwi	mango	onion
Grapefruit	avocado	papaya	squash
Cantaloupe	lemon	pear	garlic

MAY BE EATEN UNPEELED AFTER STEMS AND GREENS REMOVED AND WASHED

Plum	*tomato	**cherry**
Apricot	celery	green beans
Blueberry	bell pepper	grapes
Prunes	radish	raisins

Other packaged dried fruits

NOT ALLOWED UNLESS COOKED OR PROCESSED

Strawberry	**broccoli**	**spinach**
Raspberry	cauliflower	leafy greens
Marionberry	mushroom	lettuce
Blackberry	**cabbage**	**bulk dried fruits**

Pasteurized yogurt is allowed at all times. Avoid Nancy's, Stoneyfield, Dannon, Activia, etc.

No unpasteurized milk products; no aged cheeses (brie, bleu, sharp cheddar, etc.)

Sodas should be in cans or bottles

Nuts allowed in cans or packets, no "bulk" foods

Meats should be cooked until well done; no smoked fish

No miso or tempeh

No moldy or out-dated foods.

No "fresh" salsa or salad dressings

No home canned foods or homemade freezer jams.

OUTPATIENT

Above diet should be followed until:

Day +60 for autologous, day +100 for allogeneic (except those with active GvHD)

May go to restaurants at:

Day +30 for autologous, day +60 for allogeneic

Index

Note: The letters 'f' and 't' following locators refer to figures and tables respectively.

A

Acute coronary syndrome (ACS), 112t, 118, 181

Acute graft-*versus*-host disease (GvHD)
autologous GvHD, 184
clinical presentation, 169–170
rule of nines, 169f
evaluation and diagnosis, 170
incidence, 168
pathophysiology, 167–168
risk factors, 168
staging/grading, 170–172
findings associated with acute GvHD, 171f
Glucksberg organ staging/overall grading, 172t
steroid refractory disease, 174–184
agents for salvage therapy in steroid refractory GvHD, 175t–176t
antithymocyte globulin (ATG), 175
denileukin diftitox (Ontak®), 178
etanercept (Enbrel®), 179
extracorporeal photopheresis (ECP), 179–180
monoclonal antibodies, 180–182

mycophenolate mofetil (Cellcept®, MMF), 182
nonabsorbable corticosteroids, 182–183
pentostatin (Nipent®), 183
sirolimus (Rapamune®), 183–184
treatment, 173–174
guidelines, 173
organ specific, 174

Acute GvHD-like syndrome, 184

Acute kidney injury (AKI), 52, 248, 253–255
classification/causes/basic workup, 254–255
definitions of AKI and chronic kidney disease (CKD), 253
stages of chronic kidney disease (CKD), 254t
incidence of AKI, 254
autologous HSCT, 254
myeloablative allogeneic HSCT, 254
nonmyeloablative allogeneic HSCT, 254
renal injury, evaluation/management of causes, 255–259
calcineurin inhibitors (CNI), 258
drug toxicity, 258
marrow infusion toxicity, 257
nephrotic syndrome, 259

Acute kidney injury (AKI)
(*continued*)
sepsis, 257–258
sinusoidal obstruction
syndrome (SOS), 258
thrombotic
microangiopathy
(TMA), 258
tumor lysis syndrome
(TLS), 255–257
timing and cause of renal
injury, 255
induction therapy, 255
Acute lymphocytic leukemia
(ALL), 31t, 40t, 189,
272, 274
Acute myelogenous leukemia
(AML), 27, 31t, 40t,
189, 272–273
Acute respiratory distress
syndrome (ARDS),
235–236
Acute tubular necrosis (ATN),
254–255, 258
American Society of
Blood and Marrow
Transplantation
(ASBMT), 5–6, 121
American Society of
Hematology, 271
Angiotensin-converting
enzyme (ACE)
inhibitors, 88, 248, 268
Antibacterial prophylaxis, 76,
210
Antifungal prophylaxis,
78–79, 91, 225, 233,
283
azole dosing, 79t
Antigen-presenting cells
(APC), 83, 168
Antiplatelet therapy, 111–113
Antithrombotic guidelines

antithrombotic therapy,
113–116
atrial fibrillation, 114
CHADS2 scoring system,
115t
choice of therapy, 113
deep venous thrombosis,
116
low molecular weight
heparins, 113t
mechanical cardiac
valves, 115–116
patients developing
thrombosis, 117–118
acute coronary
syndrome, 118
catheter thrombosis, 117
deep venous thrombosis,
117
patients on antithrombotic
therapy, 111–113
antiplatelet therapy, 111
management guidelines,
112t
Antithymocyte immune
globulin (ATG), 40, 47,
94–95, 175

B
*Biology of Blood and Marrow
Transplantation*, 271
Blood and Marrow Transplant
Clinical Trial Network
(BMTCTN), 5, 263
Bone Marrow Transplant
Survivor Study
(BMTSS), 281, 289
Brain natriuretic peptide
(BNP), 247
Bronchiolitis obliterans
syndrome (BOS), 212,
233, 237–242
clinical findings, 239

definition, 239
diagnostic tests, 239–241
expiratory/inspiratory CT
    scan of chest, 240f
management, 241–242
pathogenesis of BOS, 241
risk factors, 238–239
Bronchiolitis obliterans with
    organizing pneumonia
    (BOOP), 194, 201,
    237–238, 242–243
Business of cellular therapy
    and HSCT
annual and cumulative
    transplant procedures,
    10t
common procedures with
    hospital inpatient cost,
    11t
complexity of care, 10
contract management,
    integrated structure, 14
    integrated team
    approach, 14
contracts and
    reimbursement
    strategies, 13–14
data management, 18
governmental payers, 15–16
    Medicaid, 16
    Medicare DRG
    reimbursement, 15
integrated structure for
    contract management,
    14
phases, 10–13
    harvest/acquisition, 12
    post-transplant, 12
    pre-transplant, 12
    special circumstances,
    12–13
    transplant evaluation, 10
    transplant stay, 12

private payers, 14–15
    Centers of Excellence and
    National Transplant
    Networks, 15
quality, measures, 17–18
regulatory, 16–17
    Center for International
    Blood and Marrow
    Transplant Research
    (CIBMTR), 16–17
    Food and Drug
    Administration (FDA),
    17
    Foundation for the
    Accreditation of
    Cellular Therapies
    (FACT), 16

C

Calcineurin inhibitors (CNI),
    59, 79, 93–94, 128–129,
    173, 202, 204–205, 207,
    211, 249–250, 255, 258,
    261–262, 288
Capillary leak syndrome, 44,
    178–179
Cardiovascular complications
    basic presentation/workup/
    treatment, common
    acute cardiac toxicities,
    246–249
    hypoalbuminemia, 248
    management of CHF, 248
    severe cases of CHF, 247
    tachyarrhythmias, 248
    incidence and types of
    toxicities
    occurring years following
    HSCT, 250–251
    risk factors for remote
    CHF, 250–251
    pre-transplant cardiac
    evaluation, 245–246

Cardiovascular complications
(*continued*)
  treatment-induced
    hypertension, 249–250
  posterior reversible
    encephalopathy
    syndrome (PRES), 250
Catheter thrombosis, 112, 117
Center for Disease Control
  (CDC), 64
Center for International
  Blood and Marrow
  Transplant Research
  (CIBMTR), 3, 5, 16,
  281
Center of Excellence (COE),
  15
cGvHD, therapy, 202–210
  organ-specific
    therapies/management,
    204t–206t
    eyes, 208–209
    gastrointestinal tract, 209
    hepatic, 209–210
    immunologic/infectious
      disease, 210
    lung, 209
    mouth and oral cavity,
      208
    neurologic, 210
    skin, 203
    vaginal/vulvar, 210
  systemic treatment
    strategies, 202–203
    acetretin (Soriatane®),
      203
    cyclosporine, 202
    extracorporeal photo-
      pheresis, 203
    mycophenolate mofetil
      (Cellcept®), 202
    other treatments, 203
    plaquenil, 203

prednisone, 202
    sirolimus (Rapamune®),
      202
    tacrolimus (FK 506,
      Prograf®), 202
CHADS2 scoring system, 115t
Chronic graft-*versus*-host
  (cGvHD) disease
  diagnosis and grading,
    191–196
    Clinical Trial
      Development for
      cGvHD, 196
    NIHcGHVD organ-
      specific staging form,
      197t–201t
    stigmata and clinical
      features of cGvHD,
      192t–195t
  "extensive disease,"
    definition of, 190
  follow-up, 211
  incidence and prognosis,
    189–191
    time to immune suppres-
      sion withdrawal after
      PBSC transplantation,
      190f
  "limited disease," definition
    of, 189–190
  monitoring, 196–202
    suggested studies, 196
  risk factors, 191
  syndrome of cGVHD, 189
  therapy, *see* cGvHD,
    therapy
Chronic kidney disease
  (CKD), 253–254, 258
Chronic myelogenous
  leukemia (CML), 31t,
  40t, 43, 168, 189, 272,
  274

Chronic wasting syndrome, 63

Conditioning regimens
 antiemetic dosing, 47–48
 common autologous, 40–41
 common conventional (ablative), 40
 common RIT, 40
 conditioning agents, 41–47
  antithymocytic immune globulin (ATG or ATGAM®), 41
  busulfan (Myleran®, Busulfex®), 42–43
  carboplatin (Paraplatin®), 43
  carmustine (BiCNU®, BCNU), 41–42
  cyclophosphamide (Cytoxan ®), 43–44
  cytosine arabinoside (ARA-C, Cytosar-U®), 44
  Etoposide (VP-16, Vepesid®), 44–45
  fludarabine (Fludara®), 45
  melphalan (Alkeran®), 45–46
  thiotepa (Thioplex®), 46
  total body irradiation (TBI), 46–47

Congestive heart failure (CHF), 35, 114, 245

Coronary vascular disease (CAD), 245

Corticosteroids, 90–91, 143, 157, 161, 173, 182, 202, 204, 236, 238, 241, 289

Cryptogenic organizing pneumonia (COP), 233, 238, 242–243
 clinical findings, 242
 diagnostic tests, 242–243
 management, 243

Cushing's syndrome, 135, 183

Cytomegalovirus (CMV) monitoring and preemptive therapy, 73–76

D

Deep venous thrombosis, 116–118

Diffuse alveolar hemorrhage (DAH), 78, 108, 121, 233
 clinical findings, 235
 diagnostic tests, 235
 diffuse grand ground opacities in diffuse alveolar hemorrhage, 236f
 management, 235–236
 pathogenesis, 235
 risk factors, 235

E

Encapsulated organism prophylaxis for patients with chronic GVHD, 76–78

Engraftment
 allogeneic, 120
 autologous, 119
 definitions, 119
 FACT standards for review of engraftment, 121–123
 patient/product characteristics considered in engraftment analysis, 122t
 syndrome, 120–121

Engraftment syndrome, 108, 120–121

The European Group for Blood and Marrow Transplantation (EBMT), 6, 18
Extracorporeal photopheresis (ECP), 179–180, 203

F
Fat emboli syndrome, 105
Focal segmental glomerulosclerosis (FSGS), 259
Follicle-stimulating hormone (FSH), 138, 292–293
Follow-up care
  activities of daily living guidelines, 134–135
  central venous catheters, 133–134
  diet and food preparation, 137
  endocrine assessment, 137–138
  follow-up, 125–128
    clinical evaluations, 125–126
    laboratory studies, 126–128
  immunizations, 129–133
    diphtheria-tetanus vaccine, 132
    of family members, 130
    hepatitis B vaccine, 133
    influenza, 132–133
    meningococcal vaccine, 133
    MMR vaccine, 133
    pertussis vaccine, 132
    pneumococcal vaccine, 132
    vaccination guidelines for adults post-

      autologous/allogeneic transplant, 131t
    varicella vaccines, 133
  immunosuppression, 128–129
    dose adjustment for renal insufficiency, 129t
    myeloablative transplants, 128
    nonmyeloablative transplants, 128
    renal insufficiency and calcineurin inhibitor dosing, 129
  osteoporosis, 135–137
    post-transplant factors, 136
    pre-transplant factors, 135–136
    prevention for allogeneic patients on steroid therapy, 136–137
  skin care, 137
  travel safety, 138–139
Food and Drug Administration (FDA), 17
Formal quality of life (QOL), 293
Foundation for the Accreditation of Cellular Therapies (FACT), 16, 32, 121–123
Fred Hutchinson Cancer Research Center, 188–189

G
Gastrointestinal complications
  hepatobiliary diseases, 227–230
    acute hepatitis, 229–230

gall bladder disease and pancreatitis, 230
sinusoidal obstruction syndrome or venooc-clusive disease of liver (SOS/VOD), 227–229
lower gastrointestinal, 225–227
diarrhea, 225–226
gastrointestinal bleeding, 226–227
upper gastrointestinal, 223–225
anorexia, 223–224
esophagitis/gastritis, 224–225
Gilbert's syndrome, 34
Goodpasture's syndrome, 180
Graft failure
allogeneic transplant, 266
graft rejection, 266
HLA antibody screening pre-transplant, 266–267
primary/late engraftment failure, 266
autologous transplant, 266
engraftment failure, 266
diagnosis, 267–268
bone marrow aspirate and biopsy, 267
FISH/cytogenetics, 267
peripheral blood cell counts, 267
variable number of tandem repeats (VNTR), 268
donor leukocyte infusion (DLI), 267
risk factors for graft failure, 267
treatment, 268

hematopoietic growth factors, 268
stem cell boost, 268
Graft-*versus*-host disease (GvHD) prophylaxis agents used for, 84–95
antithymocyte immune globulin (ATG), 94–95
corticosteroids, 90–91
cyclosporine and tacrolimus, 84–89
dose adjustment for renal insufficiency, 87t
methotrexate, 89–90
mycophenolate mofetil (MMF), 91–92
sirolimus, 92–94
standard regimens, 83–84
myeloablative transplant, 83
nonmyeloablative transplant, 83–84
Guillain–Barre syndrome, 180

H
Health Resources and Services Administration (HRSA), 16
Hematopoietic progenitor cell (HPC), 121–123
Hematopoietic stem cell transplantation (HSCT)
horizons/challenges, 7–8
language, 3–6
See also HSCT language, definitions
research efforts in HSCT, 6–8
chronic graft-*versus*-host disease, 8

Hematopoietic stem cell
(*continued*)
"personalized" medicine
approach, 7
Hemolytic uremic syndrome
(HUS), 88, 261–262
Herpes simplex virus
(HSV)/varicella
zoster virus (VZV)
prophylaxis, 71–73
Histocompatibility locus
antigen (HLA), 4
HSCT language, definitions
allogeneic, 4
American Society for
Blood and Marrow
Transplantation
(ASBMT), 5
autologous, 4
Blood and Marrow
Transplant Clinical
Trials Network (BMT
CTN), 5
bone marrow harvest, 5
CD34, 4
Center for International
Blood and Marrow
Transplant Registry
(CIBMTR), 5
conditioning, 5
haploidentical, 4
haplotype, 4
hematopoietic stem cell, 4
histocompatibility locus
antigen (HLA), 4
major histocompatibility
complex (MHC), 4
myeloablative, 5
National Heart, Lung,
and Blood Institute
(NHLBI), 5
National Marrow Donor
Program (NMDP), 5

non-myeloablative, 5
peripheral blood stem cell
collection (apheresis),
5
reduced intensity
transplantation, 5
syngeneic, 4
Hurler's syndrome, 30
Hypoalbuminemia, 247–248,
259

I
Idiopathic pneumonia
syndrome (IPS), 78,
233, 237–238, 237t
clinical findings, 237
diagnostic tests, 237–238
management, 238
pathogenesis of, 238
risk factors, 237
Immunizations, follow-up
care, 129–133
diphtheria-tetanus vaccine,
132
of family members, 130
hepatitis B vaccine, 133
influenza, 132–133
meningococcal vaccine,
133
MMR vaccine, 133
pertussis vaccine, 132
pneumococcal vaccine, 132
vaccination guidelines
for adults post-
autologous/allogeneic
transplant, 131t
varicella vaccines, 133
Immunosuppression,
follow-up care,
128–129
dose adjustment for renal
insufficiency, 129t

myeloablative transplants, 128

nonmyeloablative transplants, 128

renal insufficiency and calcineurin inhibitor dosing, 129

Infection prophylaxis

antibacterial prophylaxis, 76

antifungal prophylaxis, 78–79

azole dosing, 79t

cytomegalovirus (CMV) monitoring and preemptive therapy, 73–76

allogeneic patients, 73

autologous patients, 73

ganciclovir dosing in renal impairment, 75t

oral valganciclovir, 74

PCR viral load, 74

preemptive valganciclovir dosing, 74

valganciclovir dosing in renal impairment, 75t

encapsulated organism prophylaxis for patients with chronic GVHD, 76–78

herpes simplex virus (HSV)/varicella zoster virus (VZV) prophylaxis, 71–73

pneumocystis jirovecii (PCP) prophylaxis, 79–80

VRE surveillance and contact isolation procedures, 80

Infections, treatment of, 149–163

adenovirus, 155

adenovirus and BK virus infections of genitourinary tract, 153

cytomegalovirus (CMV) infection, 152

Epstein-Barr virus (EBV), 156

herpes simplex virus (HSV) infection, 151

herpes zoster infection, 149–151

dermatome map for determination of extent of herpes zoster infections, 150f

human herpes virus type 6 (HHV-6) infection, 151–152

infections with *Candida* species, 158–160

candida cystitis, 158–159

candidemia, 159–160

chronic disseminated candidiasis, 160

esophageal candidiasis, 158

invasive aspergillosis, 160–161

oropharyngeal candidiasis, 158

other fungal infections, 161–163

vulvovaginal candidiasis, 158

influenza A and B, 154–155

invasive aspergillosis, 160–161

other fungal infections, 161–163

Pneumocystis jirovecii pneumonia (PCP), 157

Infections, treatment of
(*continued*)
respiratory viral infections,
153–155
RSV, 154
Toxoplasma gondii
infection, 157–158
viral hepatitis, 156
Infectious complications
empiric antimicrobial therapy and neutropenic
fever evaluation,
145–149
criteria for removal
of central venous
catheters, 149
indications for use of
empiric extended
Gram-positive
coverage, 147–148
management of per-
sistent neutropenic
fevers, 148–149
neutropenic fever
protocol, 145–147
temporal sequence of
infections, 143–145
first month post-
transplant, 143
greater than 12 months
post-transplant, 145
1–4 months post-
transplant, 144–145
4–12 months post-
transplant, 145
phases of opportunistic
infections among
allogeneic HCT
recipients, 144f
treatment of common
infections, *see*
Infections, treatment
of

Inhibition of inosine
monophosphate
dehydrogenase
(IMPDH), 91
International prognostic
staging system ((IPSS),
29t
International Society for
Cellular Therapy
(ISCT), 121

K
Keratoconjunctivitis sicca
(KCS) syndrome, 193,
208

L
Local Coverage Deter-
minations (LCD),
15

M
Major histocompatibility
complex (MHC), 4, 83
Maturation syndrome, 41
Medicaid, 16
Medicare Coverage Database
(MCD), 15
Medicare DRG reimburse-
ment, 15
Medicare Hospital Acquired
Conditions (HAC), 16
Methicillin-resistant *Staphy-
lococcus aureus*
(MRSA), 147
Microangiopathic hemolytic
anemia (MAHA), 88,
183, 261, 263
Monitoring minimal residual
disease (MRD), 275
Multiple myeloma (MM),
24, 40t, 45, 135, 272,
274–275

Mycophenolate mofetil (MMF), 84, 91–92, 177, 182, 202, 225
Myelodysplastic syndrome, 28, 237, 300

N
National Cancer Institute Common Toxicity Criteria (NCI CTC), 5, 271, 281
National Coverage Determination (NCD), 15
National Heart, Lung, and Blood Institute (NHLBI), 5
National Marrow Donor Program (NMDP), 5, 7, 9, 18, 34, 189
National Transplant Network programs, 15
Nephrotic syndrome, 195, 259
Non-Hodgkin's lymphoma (NHL), 29–30, 40t, 275
Nutrition
explanation of catabolic/anabolic states, 67–68
tissue catabolism, 68
glutamine controversy, 68–69
ASPEN Clinical Guidelines, 68
IV glutamine, 68
oral glutamine, 69
goals of nutrition during transplant, 65–66
energy and protein requirements, 65–66
oral nutrition, 66
low-bacteria diet, 63–65
CDC guidelines, 64
water safety, 65
total parenteral nutrition, use of, 66–67
TPN administration recommendations, 67
TPN initiation guidelines, 67

O
Oral complications
discharge, 221
infections, 220
management of, 215–219
pathophysiology, 213
mucositis, 213
pre-dental procedures common regimens, 220–221
prophylaxis, 214–215
management, 217t–219t
oral hygiene during transplant, 215
oral hygiene prior to admission, 214–215
stomatitis evaluation scales, 216t
risk factors, 213–214
taste alterations, 221
Osteoporosis, follow-up care, 135–137
post-transplant factors, 136
pre-transplant factors, 135–136
prevention for allogeneic patients on steroid therapy, 136–137

P
Palliative care
core functions, direct patient care, 278–279
goal for, 278

Palliative care (*continued*)
palliative medicine,
definitions, 277–278
quality of life
continuum for
chronic/serious/advanced
disease, 280f
referral to, 279–280
Passenger lymphocyte
syndrome, 107
Peripheral blood stem cell
collection (PBSC), 25,
73, 89, 103, 106–107,
119–120, 168
mobilization
autologous transplant,
23–24
factors associated with
poor mobilization, 24
risk adapted approach,
24
strategies for hard-
to-mobilize patient,
24
Pneumocystis jirovecii (PCP),
145, 157
prophylaxis, 78–80
Posterior reversible
encephalopathy
syndrome (PRES), 250
Post-transplant relapse
allogeneic transplant recipients, considerations,
272–273
indolent/aggressive
relapse, 273
autologous transplant
recipients, considera-
tions, 271–272
lenalidomide main-
tenance therapy,
272

disease-specific treatment
for relapse, 273–275
acute lymphocytic
leukemia (ALL), 274
acute myelogenous
leukemia (AML), 273
chronic myelogenous
leukemia (CML), 274
multiple myeloma (MM),
274
non-Hodgkin's lym-
phoma (NHL), 275
future research initiatives,
275–276
mechanisms of disease
resistance, 275
molecular markers
for hematologic
malignancies, 275
pathophysiology of GvL,
275
Post-traumatic stress disorder
(PTSD), 293
Pre-transplant evaluation
allogeneic donor evalua-
tion, 36
considerations/indications,
27–30
adult acute lymphoblas-
tic/myelogenous
leukemia, 27
bone marrow failure
states, 30
chronic myelogenous
leukemia, 29
congenital
hemoglobinopathies,
30
congenital/inherited
immune disorders, 30
diffuse large B-cell lym-
phoma and aggressive

non-Hodgkin's lymphoma, 29
follicular and low-grade non-Hodgkin's lymphoma, 29
germ cell cancer, 30
mantle cell NHL, 30
multiple myeloma, 30
myelodysplastic syndrome, 28–29
pediatric acute lymphoblastic leukemia, 28
pediatric acute myelogenous leukemia, 27
cytogenetics, risk stratification for, 28t
guidelines for patient eligibility, 32–35
adequate non-hematopoietic organ function, 33
adequate performance status, 33
chemosensitive disease, 32
exclusion criteria, 34
Hematopoietic Cell Transplant Comorbidity Index, 35t
indication for transplant, 32
matched available donor/autologous stem cells collection, 34
relative contraindications, 34
hematopoietic stem cells, sources of, 31
autologous/allogeneic, 31
transplant types by disease, 31t

International prognostic index (IPI), 30t
International prognostic staging system ((IPSS), 29t
patient evaluation, 31–32
allergies and medications, 31
current disease status, 31
ECOG performance scale, 33t
family history, 32
history, 31
Karnofsky performance scale, 33t
other laboratories/testing, 32
past medical history, 31
performance status, 32
psycho-social evaluation, 32
systems evaluation, 32
Pulmonary complications
bronchiolitis obliterans syndrome (BOS), 238–242
bronchoscopy/bronchoalveolar lavage (BAL), 234
cryptogenic organizing pneumonia (COP), 242–243
diffuse alveolar hemorrhage (DAH), 234–236
idiopathic pneumonia syndrome (IPS), 237–238
See also individual entries
Pulmonary function testing (PFT), 235, 241, 243, 282, 286

R

Reduced glomerular filtration rate (GFR), 24, 253
Reduced-intensity regimens (RIT), 39–40
Renal replacement therapy (RRT), 253–255
Resource lists for survivors/ caregivers, 293t
Respiratory syncytial virus (RSV), 153–154, 234

S

Secondary malignant neoplasms (SMN), 290–291
Sinusoidal obstruction syndrome (SOS), 58, 156, 227–229, 254–255, 258
Sirolimus, 92–94
Sjögren syndrome, 208
Skin care, follow-up care, 137
Stem cell sources
  bone marrow, 22
  donor selection, 21–22
    donor screening, 22
    HLA considerations, 21–22
  peripheral blood (PBSC), 22–24
    advantages, 23
    disadvantages, 23
    largely replaced marrow, 22
    mobilization, 23–24
    target cell dose, 23
  umbilical cord blood, 25–26
    advantages/disadvantages, 25
    impact of cell dose, 25
    strategies to improve UCBT in adults, 25–26

Stem Cell Therapeutic Outcomes Database (SCTOD), 16–17
Stevens-Johnson syndrome, 179, 181
Supportive care
  acid suppression, 57
  constipation, 57
  diarrhea, 55–56
    associated with chemotherapy, 55t
  menses, 57–59
    "hormone neutral" malignancies, 58
    hormone therapy, 58
    schedule of lupron dosing, 58t
  mucositis, 56
    WHO oral mucositis grading scale, 56t
  nausea, 54–55
    anticipatory nausea, 55
    motion-induced nausea, 55
    persistent nausea, 54
    serotonin 5-HT3 inhibitors, 55
  pain management, 51–54
    PCA starting dose in opioid-naive patients, 52t
    Wong-Baker faces pain scale, 53f
  tremor, 59
Survivorship
  cardiovascular, 285–286
  endocrine, 288–289
    diabetes, 289
    hypothyroidism, 288–289
  infection, 285
  musculoskeletal complications

avascular necrosis, 290
osteoporosis, 289–290
neurologic, 287–288
cognitive dysfunction,
287
peripheral neuropathy,
288
psychosocial concerns,
293–294
pulmonary, 286–287
screening/preventive
practices for post-
transplant patients,
282–284
secondary malignant
neoplasms (SMN),
290–291
sexuality and reproductive
issues, 291–293
infertility, 291
sexual dysfunction,
292–293

T
Tachyarrhythmias, 178, 246,
248
management of, 249
Thrombotic microan-
giopathies (TM)
classification, 262
clinical presentation, 261
diagnosis, 263
Blood and Marrow
Transplant Clinical
Trial Network
(BMTCTN) Criteria,
263
International Working
Group Criteria, 263
etiology, 262–263
hemolytic uremic
syndrome (HUS),
263

risk factors, 262
thrombotic thrombocy-
topenic purpura (TTP),
263
treatment, 263–264
conditioning TM, 264
cyclosporine/tacrolimus
TM, 263–264
multi-organ fulminant,
264
systemic CMV TM, 264
Total Body Irradiation (TBI),
39, 46–48, 67, 73, 156,
235, 237, 262, 288
Total parenteral nutrition
(TPN), 57, 63, 66–67
Transfusion-associated
graft-*versus*-host
disease (TA-GvHD),
102
Transfusion medicine
day 0 transplant infusion
considerations,
105–106
cryopreserved product
infusion, 106
emergency medications,
105
marrow, 105
PBSCs, 106
transplant-associated
hemolysis, 106
peri-transplant considerations
guidelines for selecting
ABO group for
erythrocyte and
platelet-containing
components, 104t
major/minor ABO
incompatibility,
103–104

Transfusion medicine
(*continued*)
post-transplant considerations, 107–108
engraftment syndrome,
108
immune hemolysis,
107–108
pre-transplant considera-
tions, 101–102
concerns for patient with
aplastic anemia, 102
Transplant-associated thrombotic microangiopathy
(TATMA), 88, 94, 225,
254–255, 258
Travel safety, follow-up care,
138–139
Tumor lysis syndrome (TLS),
180, 255–257

U
Umbilical cord blood (UCB),
21, 25–26, 103, 125,
238

Upper respiratory tract
infection (URI), 154

V
Vancomycin-resistant
enterococcus (VRE),
147
surveillance/contact
isolation procedures,
80
Varicella zoster virus (VZV),
71, 145, 206t
seronegative immunocom-
promised allogeneic
HSCT recipients,
72

W
Wiskott-Aldrich syndrome,
30
The World Marrow Donor
Foundation (WMDA),
6

Printed by Publishers' Graphics LLC
LSI20121219.19.17.21